RECENT ADVANCES IN RHINOSINUSITIS AND NASAL POLYPOSIS

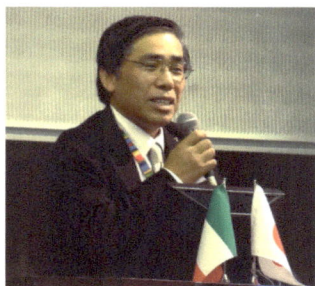
Hideyuki Kawauchi

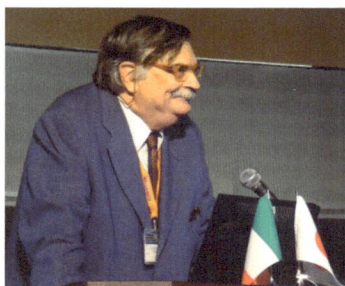
Desiderio Passali

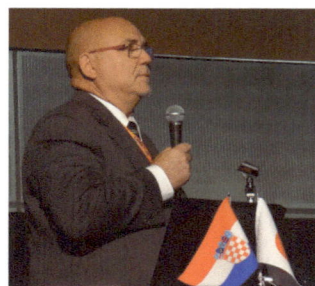
Ranko Mladina

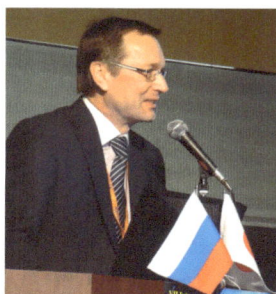
Andrey Lopatin

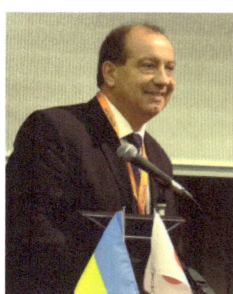
Dmytro Zabolotnyi

RECENT ADVANCES IN RHINOSINUSITIS AND NASAL POLYPOSIS

Editors

Hideyuki Kawauchi
Desiderio Passali
Ranko Mladina
Andrey Lopatin
Dmytro Zabolotnyi

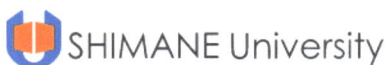

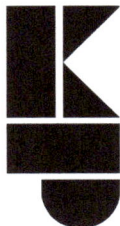

SHIMANE University

Kugler Publications/Amsterdam/The Netherlands

ISBN 13: 978-90-6299-245-4

Kugler Publications
P.O. Box 20538
1001 NM Amsterdam, The Netherlands
Telefax (+31.20) 68 45 700

website: www.kuglerpublications.com

TABLE OF CONTENTS

Table of Contents

VII International symposium on recent advances in rhinosinusitis and nasal polyposis

organized by nasal polyposis consensus group

Dates: 4-6th October, 2013

Venue: Congress Hall of Shimane Prefecture, Matsue city, Shimane, Japan

President elect: Hideyuki Kawauchi, MD,DMSc
professor and chairman,Dept of ORL,
Faculty of Medicine, Shimane University

CORRESPONDENCE
Department of Otorhinolaryngology,
Faculty of Medicine, Shimane University
89-1 Enya-cho, IZUMO city, Shimane Prefecture,
Phone: +81 853-20-2273or 2272
Fax: +81 853-20-2271
E-mail address: ISRNP7@med.shimane-u.ac.jp

PREFACE

It was my great honor and prestige to host the 7th International Symposium on Recent Advances in Rhinosinusitis and Nasal Polyposis in Matsue City, Shimane, Japan on October 4th-6th, 2013, which had been held six times before in Europe as international consensus conference on nasal polyposis. I was fortunate to welcome about 450 participants in Matsue City, including more than 100 from overseas. The three-day program aimed at inspiring participants to share updated information in this field, exchange their opinions, and prepare our future-oriented consensus report on it.

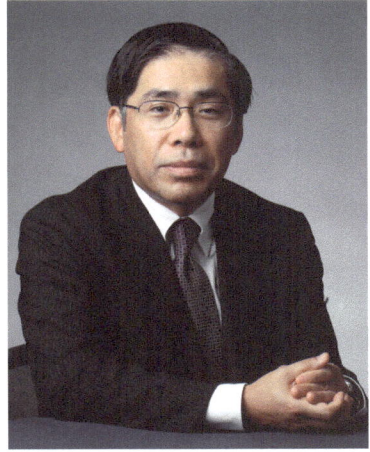

The congress opened with the Premiere Night Symposium on 'Defense System and Pathology of Respiratory Tract Inflammation' as a satellite symposium on October 3rd, being sponsored by Pacific Rim & Asian Mucin Research Symposium (PRAM), Department of Otorhinolaryngology, Shimane University, Faculty of Japan.

The opening ceremony was followed by the three-day program for researchers and clinicians, including three symposia, six workshops, six special and keynote lectures, two panels, five morning and luncheon seminars, and free oral and poster presentations.

Thanks to all delegates and volunteers, this 7th symposium was successful and had high levels of basic science and clinical investigations.

The next president elect of organizing committee for the meeting of 2015 will be prof. Amarilis Melendez, Department of Otorhinolaryngology, Edificio Royal Center, Marbella, Panama.

During the congress period, a number of overseas experts in basic science and clinical investigators with their spouses have been so generous and friendly to exchange their scientific mutual activities and private lives as well, enjoying Japanese traditional performances and meals. I would like to express my deepest appreciation to all faculty members, who enormously contributed to our scientific activities and housekeeping jobs to make this symposium a great success. I am sure that all participants enjoyed their stay in Matsue City.

To publish proceedings papers post each conference on nasal polyposis is not a tradition, but this time I decided to do so, asking many of you to submit manuscripts to make a report of what has been discussed at the 7th symposium. My cooperation with Kugler Publications, Amsterdam, The Netherlands, has resulted in publication of the proceedings as an e-book on the website of the 7th Symposium. The advantages of this e-book are that the quality is high and that all articles can be downloaded by participants free of charge. It will be usable on multiple devices: computer/laptop, tablet PCs (iPad), iPhone, e-readers, etc. It is fully searchable and has easy navigation.

If you prefer a paper copy of the actual book, Kugler Publications can also provide POD (Publishing on Demand) copies at a reasonable price. The e-book will be kept open on the web at least until the end of 2017. Hopefully, you will enjoy this e-book and utilize it as much as you can. I do believe this proceedings book will stimulate scientific research and develop clinical science as well.

Finally, I will be looking forward to seeing all of you at the 8th Symposium in Panama, very soon.

Hideyuki Kawauchi, MD, DMSc
President elect, 7th international symposium on recent advances in rhinosinusitis and nasal polyposis
Professor and Chairman, Department of Otorhinolaryngology, Faculty of Medicine, Shimane University

MANAGEMENT OF AN INVASIVE TYPE OF FUNGAL INFECTION IN PARANASAL SINUSES

N. Aoi[1], F. Takafumi[1], Y. Shimizu[1], I. Morikura[1], K. Shimizu[1], Y. Hotta[1], Q. Infei[1], E. Prokopakis[2], S. Vlaminck[3], H. Kawauchi[1]

[1]Department of Otorhinolaryngology, Faculty of Medicine, Shimane University, Izumo City, Japan; [2]Department of Otorhinolaryngology, School of Medicine, University of Crete, Crete, Greece; [3]Department of Otorhinolaryngology, School of Medicine, University of Bruges, Bruges, Belgium

Abstract

Invasive aspergillosis[1] in paranasal sinuses is not a common disease, in comparison with non-invasive type aspergillosis in paranasal sinuses. This disease usually coincides with immunocompromised hosts such as immunodeficiency patients, the aged patient, and patients with diabetes mellitus, in which cases it is called an *opportunistic infection*. The clinical outcome of these patients is often life-threatening or worse in quality of life. The prognosis varies in each case, depending on the effects of multidisciplinary treatments such as medication of anti-fungal agents and/or surgical intervention, otherwise to be fatal.

Results

We have experienced eight cases of invasive aspergillosis in paranasal sinuses, extending to the orbit and skull base[2] in the last ten years. Each case is introduced as for age, complication, disease site, beta-D-glucan in serum, symptom, bone destruction, surgical treatment, utilized anti-fungal agents, complication and prognosis (Table 1). One patient with leukemia is a 41-year-old female, the others are above 70 years of age. All of them underwent treatments involving surgical intervention combined with antifungal agents. Four patients are still alive and one of them died of another disease, three patients died of this disease in spite of the treatments.

Address for correspondence: Junichi Ishitoya, MD, PhD, Ishitoya ENT Clinic, 6-4-29-3F, Minami-karasuyama, Setagaya, Tokyo 157-0062, Japan. E-mail: ent1408@ishitoya.jp

Recent Advances in Rhinosinusitis and Nasal Polyposis, pp. 1-6
Edited by Hideyuki Kawauchi, Desiderio Passali, Ranko Mladina, Andrey Lopatin
and Dmytro Zabolotnyi
2015 © *Kugler Publications, Amsterdam, The Netherlands*

Table 1. Clinicopathological features of eight cases. Each case is introduced as for age, complication, disease site, beta-D-glucan in serum, symptom, bone destruction, surgical treatment, utilized anti-fungal agents, complication and prognosis. The patient with leukemia is a 41-year-old female; the others are over 70 years of age. All underwent treatment involving surgical intervention combined with antifungal agents. Four of the patients are still alive, the other three patients died of their disease in spite of the treatment.

	1	2	3	4	5	6	7	8
Age/Agenda	84/M	81/M	75/M	70/M	41/F	78/F	88/M	85/M
Complication	DM	Dehydration	Arrhythmia Angina	Hypertension	AML Chemotherapy	DM	DMHypertension	Lacuna infection
Sites	M	E/S	S	F	E/S	M	M	E
Fungi	*Aspergillus*	*Aspergillus*	*Aspergillus*	*Aspergillus*	*Aspergillus*	*Aspergillus*	*Aspergillus or mucor*	*Aspergillus*
βD-glucan	72.4	80	17.9	20.9	8.5	109.6	58.4	2.9
Symptom	OAS	OAS	None	Vison loss	OAS	None	OAS	Vision loss
Bony dest. (1st admin.)	Posterior	E Lateral S	Lateral	Superior	None	Orbital floor Posterior M	Posterior	None
Operation	*Caldwell-Luc*	*Killian*	*ESS*	*Killian*	*ESS*	*Caldwell-Luc*	*Caldwell-Luc*	ESS
Antifungal agent	FCZ⇒ITZ	FCZ	FCZ⇒AMPH ⇒ITZ	FCZ	FCZ⇒AMPH ⇒ITZ	MCFG⇒FCZ ⇒VCZ	L-AMB	L-AMB⇒VCZ
Orbital invasion (1st admin.)	Apex	Apex	None	Upper	Apex	Floor	Apex	None
Intracranial invasion	2 month tempo L	on adm. cavern s sur	1 month absess	on adm. dura involve	on adm. Tempo L	– –	on adm. cavern s sur	–
Outcome	DOD 93 days	DOD 22 days	DOD 120 days	DOOD 5years	alive	alive	alive	alive

OAS: orbital apex syndrome

Case presentations

We have experienced an interesting case of a 41-year-old female leukemia patient, who had complained of ptosis, visual disturbance, and headache. She was very fortunate to overcome an aspergillus infection in the ethmoid sinus with intracranial invasion, after pharmaceutical treatment with antifungal agents and endoscopic sinus surgery in the left ethmoid and sphenoid sinuses. She is still alive after a bone marrow transplantation from her daughter, combined with total body irradiation at the hematology department. The preoperative and postoperative CT scan and MRI showed findings of left ethmoid sinus and brain abscess (Fig. 1). The fungal infection subsided postoperatively. A granulomatous lesion with purulent discharge was found in the ethmoid sinus and sphenoid sinus at the operation. This lesion was carefully removed as much as possible but very conservatively to have a complete drainage from these paranasal sinuses. Case 8 is a 85-year-old male patient with left acute visual disturbance on his admission. This patient has been complaining of eye pain and visual disturbance for seven days before admission and has complications of cerebral infarction, orthostatic hypotension, and depression, but no diabetes mellitus. At admission, no abnormal finding was detected in the nasal cavity, but relative afferent pupillary defect (RAPD) is already pointed out by our out-patient

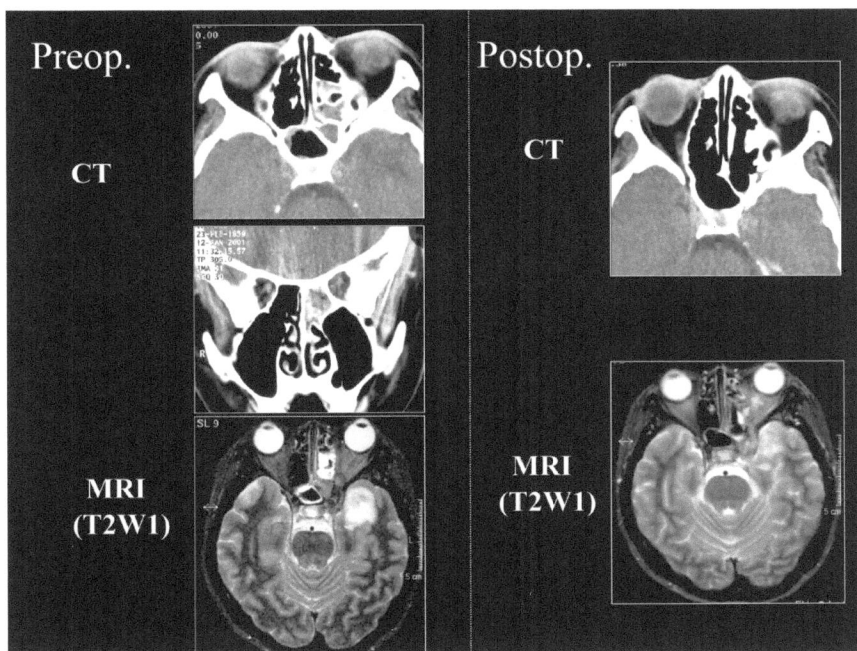

Fig. 1. The preoperative and postoperative CT scan and MRI showing findings of left ethmoid sinus and brain abscess. The fungal infection subsided after the patient received pharmaceutical treatment with antifungal agents and endoscopic sinus surgery in left ethmoid and sphenoid sinuses.

Ophthalmology clinic. Hematological examination (WBC 7,490/μl, CRP 0.11 mg/dl, β-D-glucan 2.9 pg/ml) did not indicate any remarkable fungal infection. However, MRI findings showed a nest-like structure at the orbital apex with a high signal with T1-weighted image, and a low signal with T2-weighted image, and also a high signal around the optic nerve (Fig. 2). As an invasive type of fungal infection was suspected after the MRI findings, we quickly undertook an endoscopic sinus surgery (ESS) in order to establish the fungal infection and remove the lesion. Figure 3 shows a fungus ball overlying the optic nerve

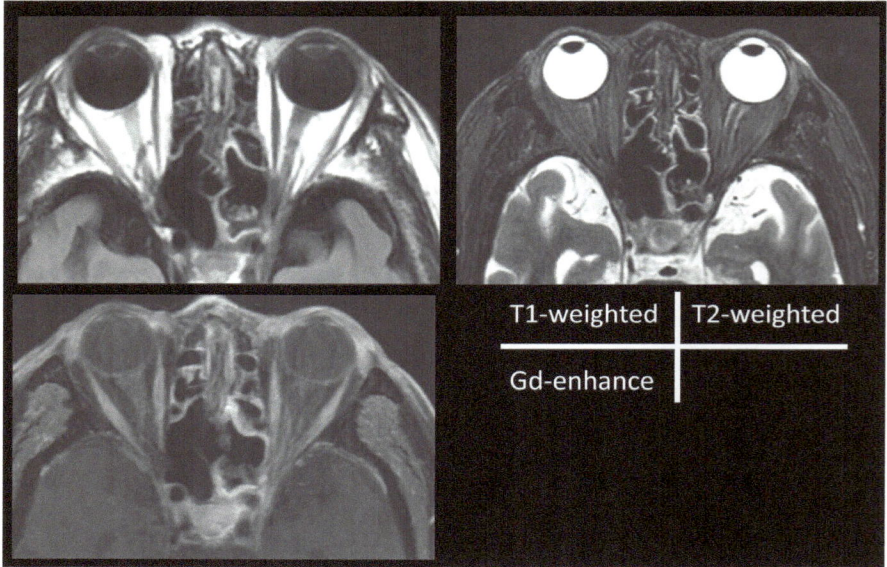

Fig. 2. Preoperative MRI findings showing the nest-like structure at the orbital apex with a high signal with T1-weighted image, and a low signal with T2-weighted image, and also a high signal around optic nerve.

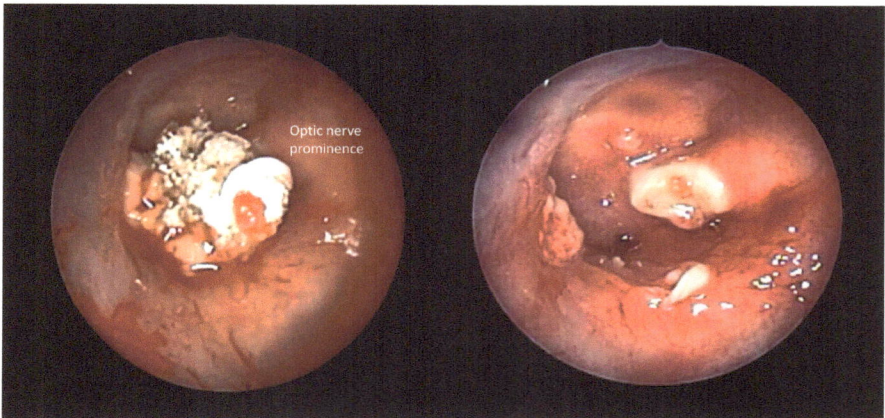

Fig. 3. Intraoperative findings of the left ethmoid sinus showing a fungus ball overlying the optic nerve prominence and exposure of inflamed optic nerve with bone destruction.

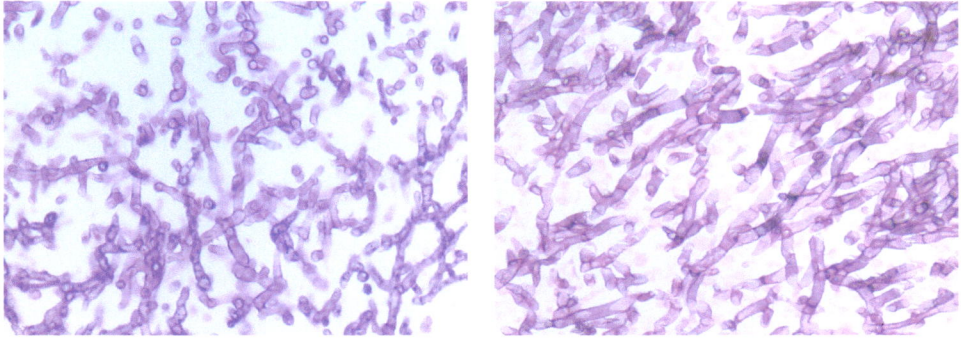

HE staining   Grocott staining

Fig. 4. Pathological findings. Hyphae were lining up, showing branching to the outer direction sharply in HE staining and septum formation was clearly shown with Grocott staining as well.

prominence and exposure of an inflamed optic nerve with bone destruction. In pathological findings (Fig. 4), hyphae were lining up, showing branching to the outer direction sharply in HE staining and septum formation was clearly shown with Grocott staining as well which proved the actual infection of *Aspergillosis* in left ethmoid sinus. Postoperatively, we performed an intensive treatment with anti-fungal agents such as L-AMB, VRCZ , and steroids. The CT finding showed neither a fungus ball nor inflammation in the ethmoid sinus, but the visual loss had not recovered yet at five months interval after ESS.

Discussion and conclusion

To summarize the case presentations, we have seen eight cases of invasive aspergillosis in paranasal sinuses, extending to the orbit and skull base. It was shown that CT scan and MRI were useful to assess the bony destruction and intracranial or intraorbital extension, respectively. The serum level of beta-D-glucan[3] and CRP was helpful for the diagnosis and monitoring of the disease activity before and after treatments. However, in three patients out of eight cases, various treatments including surgical intervention were not enough to rescue the patients and they passed away because of intracranial complication. Particularly invasive aspergillosis in paranasal sinuses can often be a fatal disease,[4] so that an earliest possible diagnosis is warranted for a better prognosis. Therefore, a clinical course in each patient should be seen to, by employing CT scan and MRI with monitoring beta-D-glucan or CRP in sera. In immunocompromised hosts, such as an aged person, diabetes mellitus, or leukemia/lymphoma patients,[5,6] a desirable radical surgical intervention is not always permitted, because of poor general condition. Taking this into consideration, very much attention should be paid to the patient's prognosis, even though the minimally invasive surgical removal of fungal lesion under ESS can be considered to be advantageous as well as a pharmaceutical treatment with antifungal agents such as liposomal AMB (empiric therapy) or voriconazole (target therapy). As for an appropriate usage of anti-fungal agents in an individual patient, the 2008 IDSA guidelines for aspergillosis, introduced by Walsh *et al.* in a clinical infectious disease journal are very useful when we have a patient with aspergillosis in different organs (Table 2).

Table 2. Recommended drugs for invasive aspergillosis (Sanford Guideline 2010).

	Fever disease (IDSA-GL refer)	*IDSA-guideline* (Walsh TJ, CID. 2008)
VRCZ (IV. PO)	Primary	A-I: Primary
L-AMB (IV)	Alternative	A-I: Alternative primary
ABLC*	Alternative	A-II Salvage
Posaconazole	Alternative	B-II:Salvage
ITCZ	–	B-II:Salvage
Caspofungin	Alternative	B-II: Salvage
MCFG	Alternative	B-II: Salvage

*ABLC: amphotericin B lipid complex

References

1. Hora JF. Primary aspergillosis of the paranasal sinuses and associated areas. Larygoscope 1965;75:768-773.
2. Smith HW, Kirchner JA, Conn NH. Cerebral mucormycosis. Arch Otolaryngol 1958;68:715-726.
3. Dupont B, Hurbor M, Kim SJ, et al. Galactomannan antigenemia and antigenuria in aspergillosis; studies on patients and experimentally infected rabbits. J Infect Dis 1987;155:1.
4. Weidenbacher M, Brandt G. Lethal aspergillosis of the paranasal sinuses. Laryngol Rhinol Otol 1975;54:722-727.
5. Hunt SM, Miyamoto RC, Cornelius RS, et al. Invasive fungal sinusitis in the acquired immunodeficiency syndrome. Otolaryngol Clin North Am 2000;33(2):335-347.
6. Malani PN, Kauffman CA. Prevention and prophylaxis of invasive fungal sinusitis in the immunocompromised patient. Otolaryngol Clin North Am 2000;33(2):301-312.

INNATE AND ACQUIRED IMMUNITY OF THE UPPER RESPIRATORY TRACT AND ITS CLINICAL IMPACT UPON THE INFLAMMATORY DISORDERS

H. Kawauchi[1], E. Prokopakis[2], N. Aoi[1], I. Morikura[1], T. Fuchiwaki[1]

[1]Department of Otorhinolaryngology, Shimane University, School of Medicine, Izumo City, Japan; [2]Department of Otorhinolaryngology, University of Crete, Crete, Greece

Introduction

It has been postulated and demonstrated that bacterial infection and its degradation products such as lipopolysaccharide (LPS) or teichoic acid (TA), induce nasopharyngeal or middle ear inflammation. Most recently, the immune reaction can be categorized as an innate immunity and acquired immunity, according to antigen specificity and various receptors on immunocompetent cells. Toll-like receptors expressed in dendritic cells, macrophages, endothelial cells, and γδT cells, play an important role in the defense mechanism against bacterial infection. On the other hand, once ostium block is achieved by mucosal swelling, paranasal sinus inflammation might become persistent. The vicious circle in middle ear cleft or paranasal sinus had been proposed and classically explained by Complement Pathway, but now it should be renewed by an updated consideration that it might be explained by interactions between bacterial degradation products and Toll-like receptors on resident epithelial cells and/or recruited inflammatory cells in there, because TLR-expressing various cells can produce and release various inflammatory cytokines or chemokines by a continuous stimulation of pathogen-associated molecular patterns (PAMPs) via Toll-like receptors.[1-4] Therefore, in this study, we have examined the role of TLRs of upper respiratory tract mucosal epithelial cells in chemokine (IL-8) and cytokine (IL-15)

Address for correspondence: Hideyuki Kawauchi, MD, DMSc, Professor and chairman, Department of Otorhinolaryngology, Shimane University, Faculty of Medicine, Izumo City, Japan. E-mail: Kawauchi@med.shimane-u.ac.jp

Recent Advances in Rhinosinusitis and Nasal Polyposis, pp. 7-13
Edited by Hideyuki Kawauchi, Desiderio Passali, Ranko Mladina, Andrey Lopatin and Dmytro Zabolotnyi
2015 © Kugler Publications, Amsterdam, The Netherlands

induction and intracellular signaling pathway, modification of inflammatory response via TLR by anti-inflammatory agents.

Materials and methods

We attempted to investigate the distribution of Toll-like receptor (TLR4 and TLR2) in upper respiratory epithelial cells such as human cell lines, by employing flowcytometry and Northern blot analysis. In an *in-vitro* study, the exact role of TLR2 and TLR4 in IL-8 and IL-15 production from upper respiratory epithelial cells was examined when these cells were stimulated with bacterial degradation products such as lipoprotein or lipopolysaccharide.

1. Cells. Human respiratory epithelial cells; CCL30,CCL185 (ATCC). Human monocyte; U937(ATCC). Medium: DMEM with 10%FCS. RPMI 1640 with 10% FCS.
2. Reagents. A-human TLR2, TLR4 and mouse IgG2a (eBioscience). Synthetic Lipid A was provided by Ono Pharmaceutics. Lipoprotein was provided by Bachem.
3. RNA analysis. Expression of TLR2, 3, 4, 6 and 9, expression of IL-15 and MyD88 was analyzed by Northern blot analysis. Total cellular RNA was prepared using TRIzol reagent. Expression of IL-15 was also analyzed by ABI 7700. IL-15 mRNA load=(value of IL-15/value of GAPDH)X104.
4. TLR2 construct: TLR2-WT is the full length epitope-tagged form of TLR2. TLR2-Δ1 and - Δ2 represent truncation of 13 or 141 amino acids at the C terminus.
5. Luciferase assay. CCL185 cells were transiently transfected with 2 mg of pGL3-NF-kB/Luc and 0.2 mg of pRL/SV40 by Lipofectamine according to the manufacturer's instruction. Twenty-four hours after the transfection, some cells were pretreated with indicated chemicals for 30 min followed by the addition of lipoprotein. After eight hours incubation with lipoprotein, cells were lysed, and the luciferase activity was measured by using the Dual-Luciferase Reporter Assay System (Toyo Ink).
6. DNA-binding assay. After 0.5 hour incubation with lipoprotein 1 mg/ml, cells were lysed. NF-kB activity was measured by using NF-kB p50 Transcription Factor Assay Kits (ACTIVE MOTIF).
7. Western blot assay: Proteins were resolved by SDS-PAGE, transferred to nitrocellulose membranes, and phosphorylation was detected by autoradiography.
8. ELISA assay. Concentration of IL-15 in the culture supernatants of respiratory epithelial cells were measured by commercial ELISA kit (GT) according to the manufacturer's instruction.

9. Flow cytometric analysis. The cells were stained with FITC-and PE conju-
gated mAb.FITC-aTLR4, PE-aTLR2mAb and mice IgG2a were used. The
stained cells were analyzed by a FACSCalibur (Becton Dickinson).
10. Statistical analysis. The statistical significance of data was determined by
Student's t-test. A value of $p < 0.05$ was taken as significant.

Results

*Distribution of TLRs in human epithelial cells in nasopharyngeal mucosae and
involvement of IL-15 in allergic reaction*

The Northern blot assay and RT-PCR data are shown in regard to TLR distribution for cultured human nasal epithelial cells, and somehow, we could not
detect any TLR4 and TLR 9 expression at messenger RNA level. As a result,
respiratory epithelial cells constitutively expressed messenger RNA for TLR2,
3, 6, but not for TLR4 and TLR9 (Fig. 1). In Northern blot analysis, IL-15
mRNA was strongly expressed after lipoprotein stimulation. In contrast, it was
not found after lipid stimulation as a ligand of TLR4. IL-15 concentration in
the supernatants of CCL185 was also upregulated after lipoprotein stimulation
in a dose-dependent manner.

Lipoprotein induced IL-15 and IL-8 production of respiratory epithelial cells,
which strictly depend on TLR2 (Fig. 2). Lipoprotein induced IL-15 production of respiratory epithelial cells was abolished by NF-kB inhibition (Fig. 3).
Lipoprotein-mediated IL-8 production in respiratory epithelial cells was abolished
with NF-kB inhibition by Oxatomide (Fig. 4).

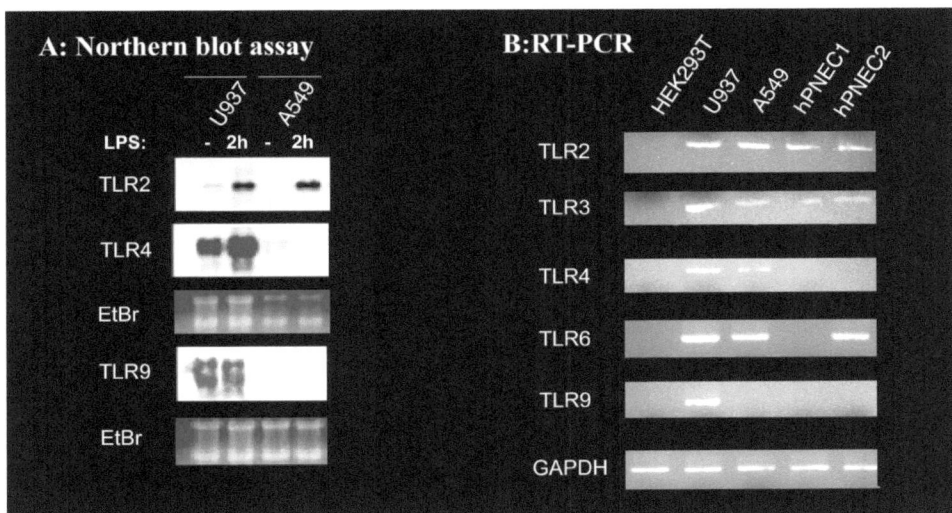

Fig. 1. Expression of TLRs on macrophages and nasal epithelial cells.

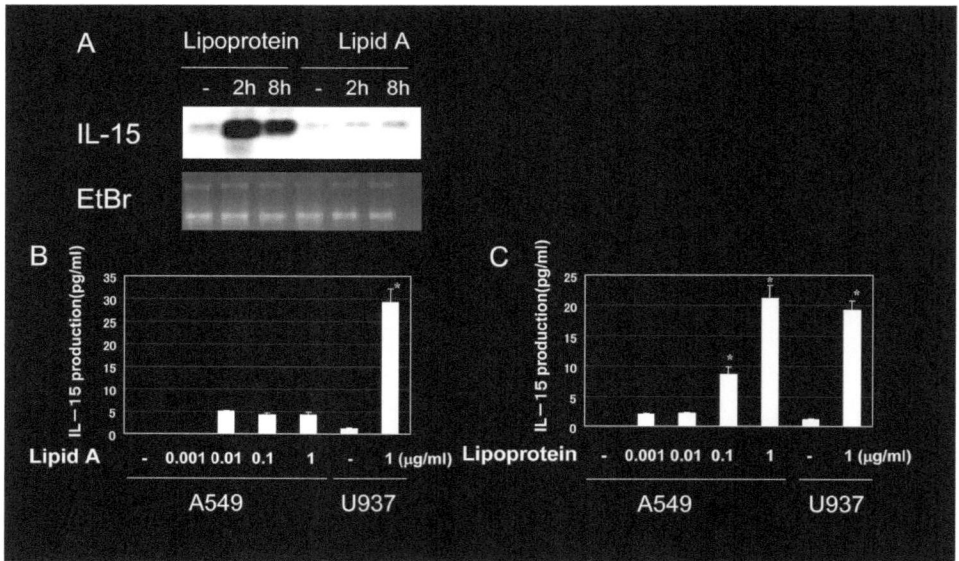

Fig. 2. Lipoprotein induces IL-15 from respiratory epithelial cells. A. Gene expression of IL-15 in A549 after lipoprotein or lipid A stimulation after Northern blot analysis. Ethidium bromide-stained gel is shown as a control. B, C. U937 and A549 cells were cultured at 1×10^6 cells/1 ml for 24 h and then in fresh medium in the absence or presence of lipid A or lipoprotein. IL-15 concentrations in the culture supernatant were determined by ELISA.

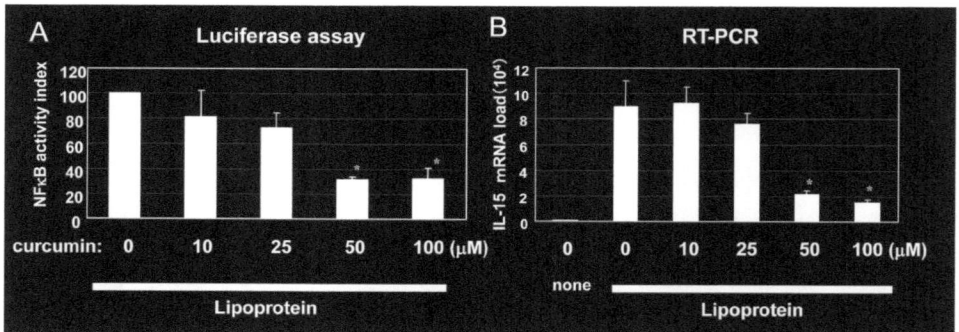

Fig. 3. Lipoprotein-mediated IL-15 mRNA induction is impaired by NF-kB inhibitor. A. Inhibition of lipoprotein-mediated NF-κB activation by curcumin in A549 cells by luciferase assay. The luciferase activity for lipoprotein treatment alone was defined as 100% in each experiment. B. Lipoprotein-mediated TLR2 mRNA increase is inhibited by a high concentration of curcumin. A549 cells were pretreated with various concentrations of cucumin for 30 min followed by a two-hour stimulation with 1 μg/ml. The gene expression of IL-15 was determined by RT-PCR.

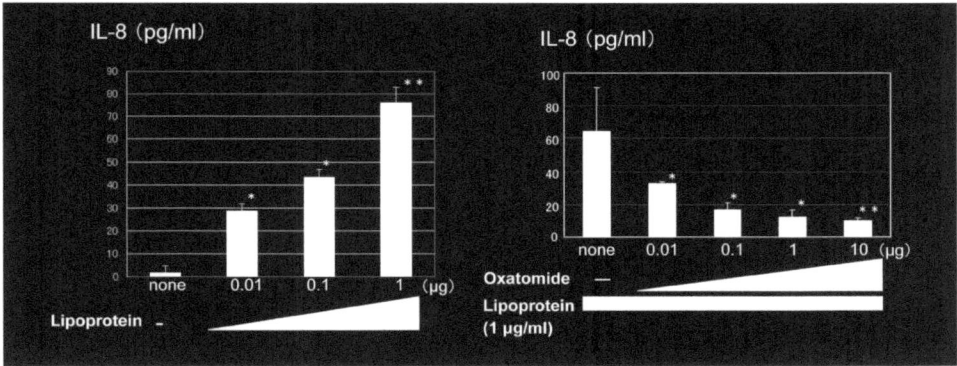

Fig. 4. Effect of oxatomide on IL-8 production in respiratory epithelial cells.

Inhibitory effect of antihistamine on cytokine production from mast cells in vitro with cross-linking with IgE and antigens

In-vitro culture of bone marrow-derived mast cells (BMMCs) indicated that allergen-induced IL-5 production from mast cells was down-regulated by Cetirizine pretreatment (Fig. 5). It was not influenced by Tranilast pretreatment. Cetilizine did not suppress IL-5 production from mast cells, if anti-DNP IgE on BMMCs was cross-linked with a high dose of DNP antigens.

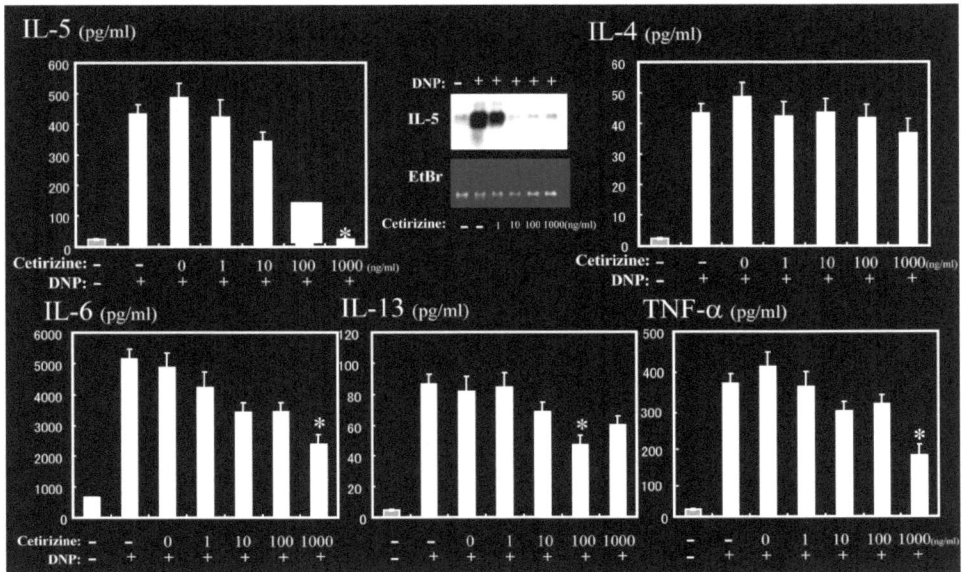

Fig. 5. Effect of Cetirizine on cytokine production from mast cells.

Effect of Lipopolysaccharide (LPS) on murine allergic rhinitis model at the eliciting phase

Mast cells, the key player at the eliciting phase of allergic rhinitis, have been reported to produce Th2 cytokines *in vitro* with LPS stimulation via TLR4 , but *in-vivo* study remains to be performed. Therefore, we investigated the LPS effect on the eliciting phase of murine allergic rhinitis model. An experimental proto- col of murine allergic rhinitis model is briefly described. At the eliciting phase, OVA antigens are intranasally introduced for seven consecutive days with LPS or without LPS, and on the final challenge, sneezing rates are counted as well as nasal tissue analysis and Th2 cytokines detected with immune-precipitation and western-blotting.

As a result, as shown in Figure 6, LPS aggravated the eliciting phase of type-I allergic reaction, in a murine allergic rhinitis model. Furthermore, the significant difference in sneezing rates between C3H/HeN mice challenged with OVA alone and OVA with LPS was found, but this difference was not detected in C3H/HeJ mice. Eosinophil infiltration was more prominent in C3H/HeN mice challenged with OVA and LPS, in comparison with those in mice challenged with OVA alone. In western blot analysis, IL-5,IL-10,IL-13 expression was seen in both groups, but IL-5 expession was upregulated in mice challenged with OVA and LPS. However, there was no significant difference in eosinophil infiltration and Th2 cytokine expression between C3H/HeJ mice challenged with OVA alone and OVA with LPS. These data taken together suggests that LPS aggravates the nasal symptom, upregulating Th2 cytokine production of mast cells via TLR4.

Discussion and future goal

In the present study, Toll-Like receptors expressed on epithelial cells, mast cells, and macrophages residing in upper respiratory tract mucosae, are demonstrated to have an important role in the pathogenesis of persistent inflammation in na- sopharyngeal cavity and middle ear cleft. Therefore, paranasal sinus or middle ear persistent inflammation might be explained by such an interaction between bacterial degradation product and Toll-like receptors on resident epithelial cells and/or recruited inflammatory cells in there. Furthermore, innate immunity is highly evaluated to non-specifically evacuate nasopharyngeal or middle ear pathogens via Toll-like receptors on epithelial cells and/or recruited inflammatory cells into the paranasal sinus or middle ear. To this end, our results may lead us to a new therapeutic strategy (H1 receptor antagonists, signal transduction inhibitors, anti-sense therapy) to down-regulate the stagnant inflammation in paranasal sinuses or tubotympanic.

References

1. Szczepański M, Szyfter W, Jenek R, et al. Toll-like receptors 2, 3 and 4 (TLR-2, TLR-3 and TLR-4) are expressed in the microenvironment of human acquired cholesteatoma. Eur Arch Otorhinolaryngol 2006;263(7):603-607.
2. McClure R, Massari P. TLR-Dependent Human Mucosal Epithelial Cell Responses to Microbial Pathogens. Front Immunol 2014;5:386.
3. Lee HY, Takeshita T, Shimada J, et al. Induction of beta defensin 2 by NTHi requires TLR2 mediated MyD88 and IRAK-TRAF6-p38MAPK signaling pathway in human middle ear epithelial cells. BMC Infect Dis 2008;8:87.
4. Moon SK, Woo JI, Lee HY, et al. Toll-like receptor 2-dependent NF-kappa-B activation is involved in nontypeable *Haemophilus influenzae*-induced monocyte chemotactic protein 1 up-regulation in the spiral ligament fibrocytes of the inner ear. Infect Immun 2007;75(7):3361-3372.

CLINICAL OUTCOME OF PATIENTS WITH INVERTED PAPILLOMA IN NASAL CAVITY AND PARANASAL SINUSES

Y. Shimizu[1], N. Aoi[1], I. Morikura[1], K. Shimizu[1], T. Fuchiwaki[1],Y. Hotta[1], E. Prokopakis[2], S. Braminck[3], H. Kawauchi[1]

[1]Dept. of Otorhinolaryngology, Shimane University, Faculty of Medicine, Izumo City, Shimane, Japan; [2]Department of Otorhinolaryngology, School of Medicine, University of Crete, Crete, Greece; [3]Department of Otorhinolaryngology, School of Medicine, University of Bruges, Bruges, Belgium

Abstract

Sinonasal inverted papilloma is a benign tumor itself , but it is not so easy to manage, because of extending occupied lesion of inverted papilloma or being combined with squamous cell carcinoma. In the last decade, we have had 31 patients actually diagnosed with sinonasal inverted papilloma. We present our management procedure and clinical outcome of patients with sinonasal inverted papilloma.

Patients and treatment protocols

The subjects were 31 patients with sinonasal inverted papilloma. The age of the patients ranged from 20 to 87 years, and the mean age was 51 years. There were 25 males and six females. The most frequent chief complaint was unilateral nasal obstruction in 24 patients, followed by nasal hemorrhage in three and postnasal drip and ocular proptosis in one. The mean duration of the symptoms reported by the patients was almost two years. Five patients visited our hospital earlier (within six months after the symptom onset), but 13 patients visited us at more than two years after the symptom onset. Our routine protocol of the diagnosis and treatment of sinonasal inverted papilloma is described here.

Address for correspondence: Hideyuki Kawauchi, MD, DMSc, Professor and chairman, Department of Otorhinolaryngology, Shimane University, Faculty of Medicine, Izumo City, Japan. E-mail: Kawauchi@med.shimane-u.ac.jp

Recent Advances in Rhinosinusitis and Nasal Polyposis, pp. 15-18
Edited by Hideyuki Kawauchi, Desiderio Passali, Ranko Mladina, Andrey Lopatin and Dmytro Zabolotnyi
2015 © Kugler Publications, Amsterdam, The Netherlands

When an easily bleeding tumor with segmented surface is noted on inspection, we perform a biopsy for pathological examination. For imaging diagnosis, CT scan, MRI, and Ga scintigraphy are carried out to establish the expanding area of the tumor and the possibility of cancer complication. For tumor markers, the serum level of SCC antigen and CYFRA21-1 are routinely examined. Surgical intervention is selected, based on the comprehensive judgement of these findings. As a therapeutic policy, we aim at complete *en bloc* excision of the lesion including surrounding healthy mucosa. For the surgical procedure, endoscopic sinus surgery, tumor resection by transmaxillary sinus approach, and/or by lateral rhinotomy are respectively performed or combined in each case.

Results

Out of the 31 patients with sinonasal inverted papilloma, biopsy for preoperative histopathological examination was performed in 20 patients, and inverted papilloma was histologically diagnosed in 19 patients. The preoperative positive rate of the pathological diagnosis was 94%. This finding suggests that preoperative histopathological examination with biopsied specimen is useful for making an appropriate treatment protocol for these patients. The preoperative serum SCC antigen and CYFRA21-1 levels in patients were also measured to consider any possible reliability for the exact diagnosis in relation with SCC complication. SCC-Ag may be a useful marker for diagnosis of this tumor as reported by other researchers. In addition, CYFRA21-1 may also serve as a useful marker for patients with cancer complication. But we should have much more cases to distinguish inverted papilloma coupled with SCC or not.

Employing the well-known Krouse's staging system of the sinonasal inverted papilloma, we examined the consistency rate of the tumor-occupied region detected by MRI before surgery, in comparison with the region confirmed during surgery. Fortunately, MRI was done for 25 patients out of 31 cases[1]. The postoperative precise pathological analysis confirmed 13 cases at stage T2, ten cases at stage T3, and two cases at stage T4, respectively. As a result, the consistency rate was 84% (21 cases out of 25) with two cases overestimation from T2 up to T3, and one case underestimation from T4 to T3. We summarized the selection of surgical procedure at our university hospital, depending upon the occupied regions in each patient. In 14 patients with stage T2, inverted papilloma advanced into the nasal cavity, extended maxillary sinus, and ethmoidal sinuses. Complication of squamous cell carcinoma was noted in three patients with stage T4. Surgical approach with lateral rhinotomy was the most frequently employed for the initial surgery in 14 patients, combined with endoscopic observation. However, non-invasive endoscopic Intranasal and sinus surgery was performed as an initial surgery in three patients. The Caldwell-Luc method and intranasal endoscopic surgery were combined in 11 patients[2-4]. The Denker method was applied to just two patients before an employment of endoscope. To see the

Table 1. Five recurrent cases of inverted papilloma. N: Nasal cavity; M: Maxillary sinus; E: Ethmoidal sinuses; F: Frontal sinus; R: Recurrence; AWD: Alive without disease; DOD: Died of disease.

Case	Age Sex	Preoperative pathological examination	Carcinoma complication	Location	Initial surgery	Additional therapy	Follow-up
1	20 Male	(-)	(-)	N	ESS (Another hospital)	LR	AWD 121 months
2	62 Male	(-)	(+)	N M E F	C-L (Another hospital)	RT > L R + SBS > R T (R)	DOD 9 months
3	60 Male	(+)	(-)	N E	ESS	D	AWD 284 months
4	62 Male	(-)	(-)	N	ESS (Another hospital)	C-L	AWD 293 months
5	52 Male	(+)	(-)	N E	LR	LR	AWD 86 months

clinical outcome of those patients, recurrence of inverted papilloma was noted in four patients, and intracranial SCC recurrence in one patient. The details of five recurrent cases are given in Table 1.

Monitoring of the tumor markers before and after the surgery is shown in Figure 1. SCC antigen levels in sera increased postoperatively only in one patient when the SCC extended into the cranium. CYFRA21-1 levels in sera increased in six patients before surgery, but decreased in all patients after surgery (Fig. 1).

Discussion

We investigated 31 patients with inverted papilloma in the nasal cavity and paranasal sinus. Twenty-four (96%) out of 25 patients were properly diagnosed preoperatively with inverted papilloma. This data suggests that preoperative histopathological examination with biopsied specimen is essential for an appropriate clinical management and better prognosis of each patient. The consistency rate of the lesion-occupied region determined by MRI was 84%, by confirming it during surgery. This finding indicates that MRI is useful for preoperative diagnosis in regard to the extension of inverted papilloma. SCC-Ag levels in sera increased in 27 of 31 patients. CYFRA21-1 levels in sera increased in six patients. The complication of squamous cell carcinoma was noted in two cases of these patients. SCC-Ag can be a useful tumor marker for diagnosis, as reported by other researchers. In addition, CYFRA21-1 may also serve as a useful marker for patients with cancer complication. Postoperative recurrence

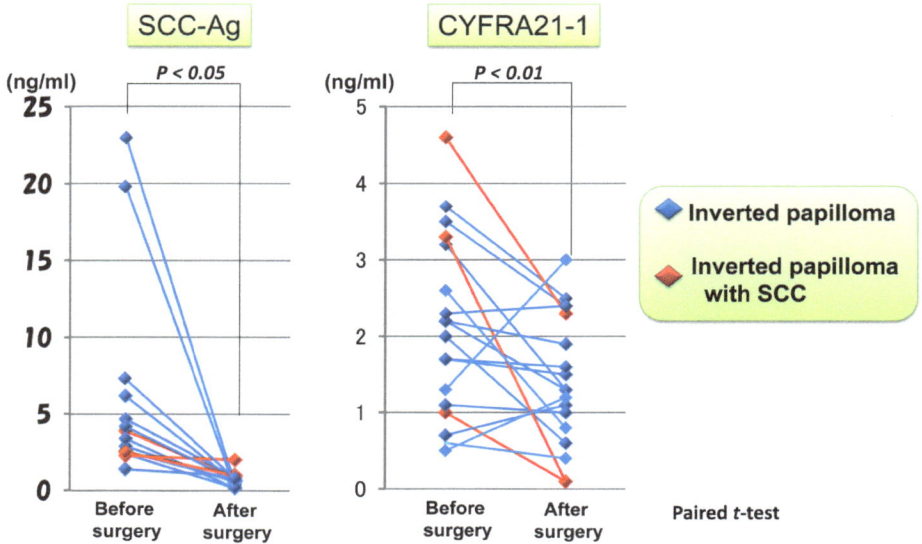

Fig. 1. Changes in the tumor markers before and after surgery.

was noted in five of the 31patients. In three of them, limited surgery had been performed without histopathological examination.

Conclusion

Our clinical data may lead us to the conclusion that in the management of patients with inverted papilloma in nasal cavity and paranasal sinuses, it is very important that we pay much attention to prepare an appropriate surgical procedure after the definite preoperative pathological diagnosis and image (CT & MRI)-guided localization of the extending tumor. Otherwise, these patients can not obtain the better prognosis.

References

1. Oikawa K, et al. Preoperative staging of sinonasal inverted papilloma by magnetic resonance imaging. Laryngoscope 2003;113(11):1983-1987
2. Sadeghi N, et al. Endoscopic removal of sinonasal inverted papilloma including endoscopic medial maxillectomy. Laryngoscope 2003;113(4):749-753.
3. Wolfe SG, et al. Endoscopic and endoscope-assisted resections of inverted sinonasal papillomas. Otolaryngol Head & Neck Surg 2004;131(3):174-179.
4. Roh HJ, et al: Tailored endoscopic surgery for the treatment of sinonasal inverted papilloma. Am J Rhinol 2004;18(2):65-74.

THE ROLE OF HMGB1 PROTEIN IN CRS WITH/ WITHOUT NP PATHOPHYSIOLOGY

L.M. Bellussi[1], J. Cambi[1], F.M. Passali[1], D. Passali[1]

[1]ENT Department, University of Siena, Siena, Italy; [2]ENT Department, 'Tor Vergata' University, Roma, Italy

Introduction

The respiratory system is regularly exposed to altered environmental conditions as well as constantly bombarded by environmental pollutants, respiratory pathogens, and aerosolized toxins. Thus, the system has evolved multiple physiologic strategies to regulate inspired air flow resistance, temperature, and humidification, as well as tightly modulate its ability to protect and defend itself. Disruption of these physiologic processes secondary to host or environmental factors such as anatomic variations, genetic mutations, overwhelming environmental pollution, or frequent infections contribute to the development of chronic rhinosinusitis.

The barrier function of nasal epithelium is a new concept developed in the last decade.[1]

Intrinsic host deficits in nasal epithelium results in reduced production of innate immune anti-microbial molecules. Local immune deficits allow the colonization and overgrowth of microbial agents. Microbial agents are capable of activating epithelial cells through pre-programmed pathways. The integrity of the epithelial barrier is disrupted secondary to epithelial activation, pro-inflammatory factors release and deregulation of the local inflammatory microenvironment .

The airway epithelium acts as a frontline defense against respiratory viruses, not only as a physical barrier and through the mucociliary apparatus but also through its immunological functions.

The interaction between respiratory viruses and airway epithelial cells results in production of antiviral substances, including type I and III interferons, lactoferrin, β-defensins, and nitric oxide, and also in production of cytokines and chemokines, which recruit inflammatory cells and influence adaptive immunity.[2]

Address for correspondence: Luisa M. Bellussi MD, ChD ENT Department, Università di Siena, Viale Bracci, 16 53100, Siena, Italy. E-mail: l.bellussi@virgilio.it

Recent Advances in Rhinosinusitis and Nasal Polyposis, pp. 19-27
Edited by Hideyuki Kawauchi, Desiderio Passali, Ranko Mladina, Andrey Lopatin and Dmytro Zabolotnyi
2015 © Kugler Publications, Amsterdam, The Netherlands

The airway epithelium is at the interface of the human body with the inhaled environment and forms a complex physicochemical barrier complemented by the mucociliary escalator to provide the first line of defense against inhaled pathogens (mechanical barrier).

Mucus overlying the airway epithelium provides further protection of the mucosa by creating a semipermeable barrier that enables the exchange of nutrients, water, and gases while being impermeable to most pathogens (physicochemical barrier).

Innate immune responses of the epithelium allow for control of viral invasion and replication, and adaptive responses allow for effective viral clearance through cells of the adaptive immune system. Airway epithelial cells rapidly recognize pathogens through pattern recognition receptors (PRRs) such as toll-like receptors (TLRs) and intracellular viral sensors (innate immunity barrier).

TLRs are type I integral membrane glycoproteins which recognize a variety of pathogen-associated molecular patterns (PAMPs). In mammals, 13 members of the TLR family have been identified so far.[4]

The innate immune system is activated also by endogenous danger signals, *i.e.*, endogenous peptides constitutively present in granules of leukocytes or epithelial cells and released from damaged and necrotic cells.

Together with PAMPS, these peptides constitute the big family of damage-associated molecular patterns (DAMPs) representing the first host response to exogenous (infections) and endogenous (injuries) danger signals.

Tight junctions (TJs) reside immediately below the stratum corneum and regulate the selective permeability of the paracellular pathway interacting with protein-receptor system.

Claudin-1 plays a critical role in human epidermal TJ function and keratinocyte proliferation. Expression of Claudin-1 is significantly reduced in non-lesional skin of patients with atopic dermatitis compared with non-atopic subjects and patients with psoriasis. Claudin-1 levels are inversely correlated with TH2 biomarkers, suggesting that reductions in this key TJ barrier protein might affect the character of the immune response to environmental allergens.[4]

A decreased trans-tissue resistance was found in biopsy specimens from patients with CRS with nasal polyps along with an irregular, patchy, and decreased expression of the TJ molecules occludin and zonula occludens 1. Trans-epithelial resistance (TER) was reduced in air-liquid interface cultures from patients with CRS with nasal polyps. The cytokines IFN-γ and IL-4 decreased TER, whereas IL-17 did not have any influence on epithelial integrity.

The disruption of epithelial integrity by IFN-γ and IL-4 *in vitro* indicates a possible role for these pro-inflammatory cytokines in the pathogenesis of patients with CRS.[5]

Surfactant proteins, SP-A and SP-D, are collagen-containing C-type (calcium-dependent) lectins called collectins and are involved in viral neutralization, clearance of bacteria, fungi, apoptotic and necrotic cells, down regulation of allergic reaction and resolution of inflammation.

SP-A and SP-D can bind various self and non-self ligands, while the collagen region can recruit and activate the immune cells for the clearance of pathogens and apoptotic/necrotic cells. In addition to anti-microbial activities, SP-A and SP-D also play an important role in the control of inflammation triggered by self, non-self and altered self cells and molecules. Thus, they have a pivotal role in the clearance of apoptotic and necrotic cells, dampening of allergic reactions, maintenance of pregnancy (by virtue of their presence in the amniotic fluid), and modulating dendritic cell (DC) and T cell properties.[6]

SP-A suppresses the allergen-induced inflammation enhancing the uptake of apoptotic eosinophils; it has a role in binding pollens grains in asthmatic patients; increasing membrane permeability it inhibits P. aeruginosa growth and gives rise to H. influenzae aggregation and opsonization.

SP-D binds and inhibits viruses; decreases eosinophils migration; increases membrane permeability and so inhibits fungal pathogens.

HMGB1

HMGB1 in homeostatic conditions is a non-histonic DNA-binding protein,[7] but when released extra-cellularly, it plays the role of potent pro-inflammatory cytokine.[8]

Extracellular HMGB1 binds to different membrane receptors (TLR2, TLR4, RAGE) and through activation of the transcriptional factor Nuclear Factor kB (NF-kB) causes the release of pro-inflammatory mediators, cytokines and chemokines, it induces endothelial activation and increases survival of inflammatory cells, mainly eosinophils.[9]

Low levels of HMGB1 usually mediate beneficial responses in reaction to environmental or endogenous dangers, enhancing both the innate and adaptive immune system and promoting inflammation and tissue repair. High levels cause acute damage: its binding to RAGE receptor expressed by endothelial cells, promotes the recruitment of inflammatory cells – especially eosinophils –- their survival and release of inflammatory mediators such as ECP and MBP from these cells with subsequent epithelial barrier damage.

There is an active release of HMGB1 for example from activates eosinophils with immunostimolatory effects, and a passive release by necrotic epithelial cells. HMGB1 interact with NF-kB[10] a nuclear transcription factor more expressed in nasal polyposis (NP). NF-kB can induce the transcription of cytokines, chemokines and adhesion molecules, which play an important role in the inflammatory process. Moreover, transcription factors influence the response to corticosteroids, which are the basis of NP treatment.

Pathological effects

HMGB1 protein has been shown to play a role in the pathogenesis of several inflammatory diseases, such as hepatitis, arthritis, stroke, liver and kidney ischemia, sepsis,[11] rheumatoid arthritis[12] and systemic lupus erithematosus.[13]

Personal experiences

Our recent researches were addressed to investigate the HMGB1 role in the pathogenesis of chronic nasal mucosa inflammatory diseases such as allergic rhinitis, chronic rhinosinusitis and nasal polyposis.

The aims of our first study[14] were (1) to determine whether HMGB1 is augmented in chronic rhinosinusitis with nasal polyps (CRSwNP); (2) if its expression is associated with eosinophils, TNF-α, IL5 and IL8, cytokines typically present in chronic inflammation of the nose and paranasal sinuses; (3) to investigate a hypothetical role of this protein in the pathogenesis of nasal polyposis. For this purpose, nasal polyps tissue from 21 patients with CRSwNP including one patient with asthma and two patients with allergic rhinitis, and eight healthy control subjects were collected. CRSwNP was confirmed by medical history, nasal endoscopy and computed tomography (CT). Control subjects were patients with rhinorrhoea of cerebrospinal fluid, fracture of the optic canal or a benign skull base tumor and did not have a history of sinus disease or asthma.

Biopsy specimens of nasal mucosa and nasal polyps were collected before surgery. Samples were subjected to haematoxylin-eosin (HE) staining and immunohistochemistry to investigate HMGB1 protein expression and its correlation with eosinophils and IL-5, IL-8 and TNF-α cytokines. Part of the fresh tissue was snap-frozen at -180° for immunohistochemical staining.

According to HE staining, subjects were divided into three groups: eight control subjects, ten eosinophilic CRSwNP patients and 11 non-eosinophilic CRSwNP patients.

Expression of HMGB1 in inflammatory cells in patients with both eosinophilic and non-eosinophilic CRSwNP was significantly increased compared to the controls. HMGB1 protein was increased in the nucleus of epithelial cells, or as focal subepithelial infiltration and in inflammatory cells independently from the aetiologic stimuli (Fig. 1). Our research suggested that HMGB1 may play a crucial role in the pathogenesis of chronic rhinosinusitis with nasal polyps and IL-5, IL-8 and TNF-α positive cells might be involved in the regulation of HMGB1.

Differing from white patients, Chinese and Japanese CRSwNP patients display different patterns of sinus mucosal inflammation[15] and more than one-half of CRSwNP patients in our sample presented neutrophilic CRSwNP.

'Eosinophilic chronic rhinosinusitis' (ECRS) was introduced to identify a subgroup of chronic rhinosinusitis which is different from non-ECRS in terms of many clinical features: symptom appearance, occurrence site of nasal polyps, CT scan findings, the histology of nasal polyps, blood examination findings, clinical course after surgery, and co-morbid asthma, etc.

In a subsequent study[16] the expression levels of HMGB1 protein in Chinese patients with CRSwNP with or without eosinophilia were investigated. Immunostaining results demonstrated that nasal polyps specimens with different endotypes had different expression levels of HMGB1 in the nucleus predominantly, as well as in the cytoplasm. Analyzing the messenger RNA (mRNA) levels of HMGB1,

Immunohistochemical staining results

Normal   Eos CRSwNP   Non-Eos CRSwNP

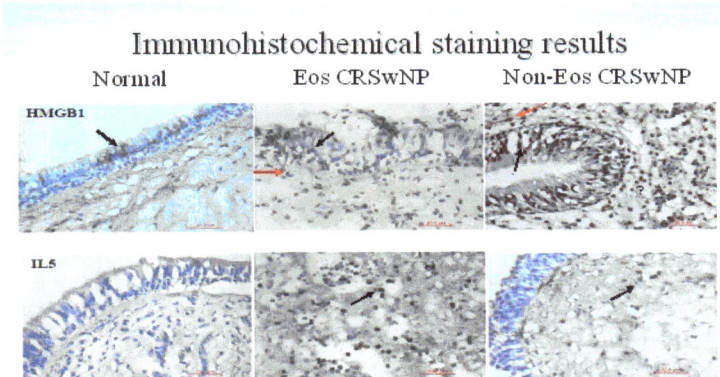

Fig. 1. Immunohistochemical staining for HMGB1 and IL-5 (X40). Immuno-localization of HMGB1 in nasal polyposis. Immuno-histochemical staining revealed that HMGB1 protein is detectable in controls, but the staining is more evident in patients with CRSwNP, and it is expressed in the nucleus and cytoplasm. IL-5 is detectable in the sub-epithelial layer of patients with CRSwNP. Black arrows show HMGB1 expression in epithelial cells, while red arrows show focal infiltration in sub-epithelial layers. (From: Bellussi L. et al. 2012[14])

IL-5, IL-8, and TNF-α, they were significantly higher in eosinophilic CRSwNP than those from controls and non-eosinophilic CRSwNP, and no significant differences in these markers were found between non-eosinophilic CRSwNP and controls. HMGB1 expression levels correlated significantly and positively with IL-5, IL-8, and TNF-α ($rs = 0.665, 0.771$, and 0.724, respectively; $p < 0.001$) and slightly with eosinophil infiltration ($rs = 0.149$; $p = 0.012$) and the blood eosinophils count ($rs = 0.225$; $p = 0.001$) in all samples.

Thus HMGB1 protein has a role in the pathophysiology of ECRS: together with IL-5, IL-8, and TNF-α may form a pro-inflammatory loop promoting chronic inflammation of nasal and paranasal sinus mucosa and NP and the eosinophilia classification together with higher HMGB1 expression may be a better defining subgroup than 'polyps/no polyps'.

Another study[17] was aimed at confirming the role of HMGB1 in NP and CRS, and at investigating if its expression and localization (nuclear, cytoplasmic, extracellular) is, in the same way, related to the severity and complexity of the histological and clinical picture.

With this aim, ten biopsies of nasal mucosa from patients with CRS without NP and 31 CRS with NP were randomly selected; as controls three biopsies of normal nasal mucosa harvested from healthy patients with no symptoms of chronic rhinosinusitis or nasal allergies were included. No inflammatory infiltrate, fibrosis, neoformation of vessels or eosinophils were found by the pathologist in these specimens.

Patients' assessment was based on clinical history, symptoms collection and severity evaluation, presence or absence of allergy, asthma, ASA intolerance, other allergic manifestations (drug allergy), previous surgery, recurrences.

The tissue samples were tested by immunohistochemistry (IHC) using HMGB1 polyclonal antibody and thereafter counterstained with Meyer's hematoxylin. The biopsy samples were analyzed with two different aims: the first aim was to evaluate the HMGB1 expression and its cellular distribution. For this purpose, nuclear, cytoplasmic and extracellular staining was estimated as a percentage of the total staining in the examined area and the intensity of HMGB1 positivity was classified according to the percentage. The second aim was to compare this distribution with the inflammatory infiltrate and the severity of the clinical picture.

As expected, all the patients with a higher inflammatory infiltrate and eosinophils presence had an allergic-hyperreactive condition or co-morbidity, that may induce and sustain the nasal mucosa inflammation. We investigated the correlation of eosinophils presence and nuclear HMGB1 values, and we noticed decreased nuclear levels in patients with eosinophils absence and increased levels in patients with higher eosinophils scores.

Since according to our hypothesis, HMGB1 might be a marker of certain disease activity, we evaluated allergic patients and non-allergic patients for the presence of HMGB1: we found a statistical significance for extracellular HMGB1 and nuclear HMGB1, both increased in allergic patients. The presence of other allergic-hyperactive conditions such as asthma, NSAIDs (non-steroidal anti-inflammatory drugs) intolerance, antibiotic allergy was additionally assessed on HMGB1 levels. The results obtained were interpreted as a statistical significance between extracellular HMGB1 and NSADs intolerance; around statistical significance for antibiotic allergies and nuclear HMGB1. The higher extracellular HMGB1 expression in patients with more severe clinical and inflammatory pictures and the presence of associated co-morbidities confirms the role of HMGB1 in the induction of the inflammatory reaction and evidences its importance for the process becoming chronic.

As a whole, these results are particularly interesting if red in the light of the inflammatory/anti-inflammatory mechanisms. Indeed, the pharmacological research could be addressed to seek for new compounds which, decreasing the extra-cellular levels of this protein by a scavenger mechanism, could keep under control the inflammatory process without interfering with the nuclear transcriptional messengers and blocking, at the same time, the feedback loop which characterizes the HMGB1 mechanism of action.

To better understand the pathophysiological role of HMGB1 in inflammation, we performed an '*in-vitro*' experimental study[18] using primary cultures of human nasal epithelial (HNE) cells, and following the lipopolysaccharides (LPS) induced active translocation and release of HMGB1 by immunofluorescence assay and Western blot.

We obtained epithelial cells of nasal polyps and paranasal sinus mucosa from ten patients requiring surgery for their sinusitis, excluding cases with non-invasive fun-gal sinusitis, chronic obstructive pulmonary disease, cystic fibrosis, primary ciliary dyskinesia (PCD) or severe asthma.

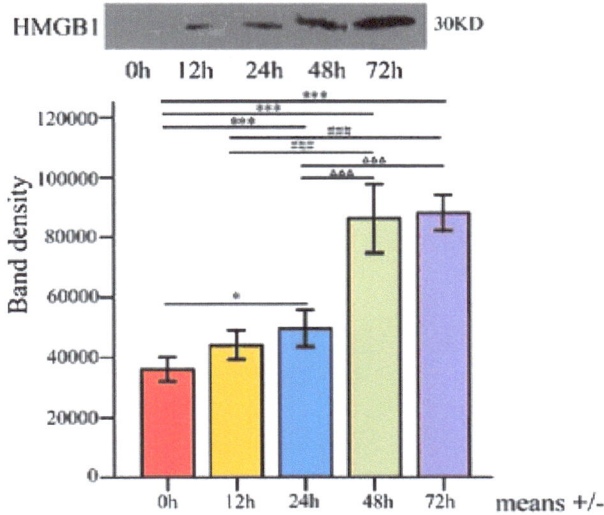

Fig. 2. HMGB1 expression in epithelial cells. Levels of released HMGB1 from HNE cells exposed to 100 µg/ml LPS from 0 hr to 72 hr by Western blot analysis. *p < 0.05; ***p < 0.001; ###p < 0.001; p < 0.001. (From: Chen D. et al. 2013[18])

Escherichia coli LPS was added during mucociliary differentiation at the working concentrations of 10 µg/ml, 50 µg/ml and 100 µg/ml. The levels of HMGB1 protein in epithelial cells and supernatants were assessed after 0, 12, 24, 48 and 72 hr by Western blot.

The study documented for the first time the presence of HMGB1 immuno-staining in the nuclei of HNE cells from nasal polyps thus confirming our hypothesis that HNE cells should be considered active participants of the innate immunity mechanisms: after LPS stimulation, translocation of HMGB1 from nuclei to cytoplasm occurred, suggesting that HNE cells represent a potential source of the secreted form of HMGB1 in the airways.

This finding was in agreement with the results of Western blot analysis: in fact, the level of intracellular HMGB1 protein did not change in the early stages (0-24 hr) of stimulation, but increased significantly at 48 hr and maintained a higher level for up to 72 hr (Fig. 2).

At the same time, secreted HMGB1 in the cultured supernatant of the LPS-treated HNE cells was detectable after 12 hr, and the concentration of HMGB1 significantly increased at 24 hr after onset of treatment and continued to increase steadily.

As a whole, our findings suggest that HMGB1 plays an important role in the induction and prolongation of the mechanisms of infection or injury-elicited inflammatory response of HNE cells.

All our studies suggest that HMGB1 inhibition might be an efficacious and innovative therapeutic target for patients with chronic upper airways and nasal mucosa inflammatory diseases.[13]

HMGB1 inhibition could be obtained by three main strategies:
1. Blocking HMGB1 release by necrotic cells and activated immune cells. This is a disadvantageous mechanism because it suppresses the protein physiological homeostatic function in all cells with serious side effects.
2. Blocking RAGE, TLR2, TLR9 receptors with antagonist drugs. This mechanism is risky because HMGB1 receptors also mediate other immune effects, such as the antibacterial activity.
3. Inactivating HMGB1 after its release: this strategy is currently the most effective and safest.

Among the molecules that bind HMGB1 there is glycyrrhizin, a glycoside alkaloid present in large quantities in Glicyrrhiza glabra roots, the plant from which licorice is extracted.[19]

Glycyrrhizin is composed of a molecule of glycyrrhetic acid (the active component of the molecule) and two molecules of glucuronic acid.

The glycyrrhetic acid inhibits the HMGB1 chemotactic and mitogenic function binding to the hydrophobic residues that delimit the pockets in Box A and B, without significant distorting their secondary structure and hence without impeding the ability of DNA binding.[20]

Several studies show the absence of cytotoxicity even at high concentration and good pharmacological tolerability of glycyrrhizin both in rats and in humans.[21]

With this background, recent studies have evaluated the potential therapeutic effects of glycyrrhetic acid in ENT diseases, particularly allergic rhinitis in children.[22,23]

References

1. Fokkens WJ, Lund VJ, Mullol J, et al. EPOS 2012: European position paper on rhinosinusitis and nasal polyps 2012. A summary for otorhinolaryngologists. Rhinology 2012;50:1-12.
2. Vareille M, Kieninger E, Edwards MR, Regamey N. The airway epithelium: soldier in the fight against respiratory viruses. Clin Microbiol Rev 2011;24:210-229.
3. Kumar H, Kawai T, Akira S. Toll-like receptors and innate immunity. Biochem Biophys Res Commun 2009;388:621-625.
4. De Benedetto A, Rafaels NM, McGirt LY, et al. Tight junction defects in patients with atopic dermatitis. J Allergy Clin Immunol 2011;127:773-86.e1-7.
5. Soyka MB, Wawrzyniak P, Eiwegger T, et al. Defective epithelial barrier in chronic rhinosinusitis: the regulation of tight junctions by IFN-γ and IL-4. J Allergy Clin Immunol 2012;130:1087-1096.e10.
6. Nayak A, Dodagatta-Marri E, Tsolaki AG, Kishore U. An Insight into the Diverse Roles of Surfactant Proteins, SP-A and SP-D in Innate and Adaptive Immunity. Front Immunol 2012;3:131.
7. Verrijdt G, Haelens A, Schoenmaker E, Rombauts W. Claessen Comparative analysis of the influence of the high-mobility group box 1 protein on DNA binding and transcriptional activation by the androgen, glucocorticoid, progesterone and mineralcorticoid receptors Biochemistry Journal 2002;361:97-103.
8. Scaffidi P, Misteli B, Bianchi ME. Release of chromatin protein HMGB1 by necrotic cells triggers inflammation Nature 41 2002;191-5.

9. Bianchi ME, Manfredi AA. High-mobility group box 1 (HMGB1) protein at the crossroads between innate and adaptive immunity. Immunol Rev 2007;220:35-46.
10. Valera FC, Queiroz R, Scrideli C, Tone LG, Anselmo-Lima WT. Expression of transcription factors NF-kappaB and AP-1 in nasal polyposis. Clin Exp Allergy 2008;38:579-585.
11. Wang H, Bloom O, Zhang M, et al. HMG-1 as a late mediator of endotoxin lethality in mice. Science 1999;285:248-251.
12. Wittemann B, Neuer G, Michels H, Truckenbrodt H, Bautz FA. Autoantibodies to non-histone chromosomal protein HMG-1 and HMG-2 in sera of patients with juvenile rheumatoid arthritis. Arthritis Rheum 1990;33:1378-1383.
13. Ayer LM, Rubin RL, Dixon GH, Fritzler MJ. Antibodies to HMG proteins in patients with drug-induced autoimmunity. Arthritis Rheum 1994;37:98-103.
14. Bellussi LM, Chen L, Chen D, Passali FM, Passali D. The role of high mobility group box 1 chromosomal protein in the pathogenesis of chronic sinusitis and nasal Polyps. Acta Otorhinolaryngol Ital 2012;32:386-392.
15. Ishitoya J, Sakuma Y, Tsukuda M. Eosinophilic chronic rhinosinusitis in Japan. Allergol Int 2010; 59:239-245.
16. Chen D, Mao M, Bellussi LM, Passali D, Chen L. Increase of high mobility group box chromosomal protein 1 in eosinophilic chronic rhinosinusitis with nasal polyps. Int Forum Allergy Rhinol 2014;4:453-462.
17. Bellussi LM, Iosif C, Sarafoleanu C, et al. Are HMGB1 protein expression and secretion markers of upper airways inflammatory diseases? J Biol Regul Homeost Agents 2013;27:791-804.
18. Chen D, Bellussi LM, Passali D, Chen L. LPS may enhance expression and release of HMGB1 in human nasal epithelial cells in vitro. Acta Otorhinolaryngol Ital 2013;33:398-404.
19. Mollica L, De Marchis F, Spitaleri A, et al. Glycyrrhizin binds to high-mobility group box 1 protein and inhibits its cytokine activities. Chem Biol 2007;14:431-441.
20. Ploeger B, Mensinga T, Sips A, et al. The pharmacokinetics of glycyrrhizic acid evaluated by physiologically based pharmacokinetic modeling. Drug Metab Rev 2001;33:125-147.
21. van Rossum TG, Vulto AG, Hop WC, et al. Intravenous glycyrrhizin for the treatment of chronic hepatitis C: a double-blind, randomized, placebocontrolled phase I/II trial. J Gastroenterol Hepatol 1999;14:1093-1099.
22. Mansi N, D'Agostino G, Scire AS, et al. Allergic Rhinitis in Children: A Randomized Clinical Trial Targeted at Symptom. Indian J Otolaryngol Head Neck Surg 2014;66:386-393.
23. Salpietro C, Cuppari C, Grasso L, et al. Nasal high mobility group box 1 protein in Children with allergic rhinitis. Int Arch Allergy Immunol 2013;161:116-21.

THE NEW ASPECTS OF POLYP FORMATION

D. Zabolotnyi, S. Yaremchuk

SI Institute of Otolaryngology Prof. O.S. Kolomiychenko, National Academy of Medical Sciences of Ukraine, Kiev, Ukraine

The prevalence of chronic inflammatory and allergic diseases of the upper airways showed an upward trend over the past 30 years, particularly in industrialized countries. One of the reasons for this increase is the pollution of the environment by substances that contain estrogens, as well as xenoestrogens. These chemical substances are present in herbicides, pesticides, detergents and plastics. By getting into the drinking water or having a close contact with the skin and mucous membranes, they react with estrogen receptors and stimulate them.

Besides xenoestrogens, there are also phytoestrogens that have high affinity with the receptors and exhibit estrogen-like action. As a result, this reaction leads to the malfunction not only in the sexual sphere, but also in other organs and systems where the estrogen receptors are located.

But first, a few words about the history of research of estrogen receptors. In 1986, E. Parfenova found receptors of estradiol in rat's nasal mucosa. In 1987, V. Bikov showed that estrogen disbalance leads to disorders of the maturing of epithelium and promotes fungi adhesion. In 1994, X. Zhao stated that levels of estrogen might have different effects on the nasal mucosa. In 2003, Jan-Ake Gustafsson discovered two types of estrogen receptors: estrogen receptor (ER)-α and ER-β.

Through these receptors, estrogens carry out management in organism; ER-α often exerts an activating function and accelerates various processes, including cell division. ER-α activity is mainly aimed at regulating fertility and conception. ER-β has the opposite effect, retarding processes such as cell division and simulating cell death (apoptosis).

Address for correspondence: D. Zabolotnyi, SI "Institute of otolaryngology of Prof. O.S. Kolomiychenko, National Academy of Medical Sciences of Ukraine", Zoologichna st.3, Kiev 03057, Ukraine. E-mail: yaremchuk@mail.ru

Recent Advances in Rhinosinusitis and Nasal Polyposis, pp. 29-31
Edited by Hideyuki Kawauchi, Desiderio Passali, Ranko Mladina, Andrey Lopatin and Dmytro Zabolotnyi
2015 © Kugler Publications, Amsterdam, The Netherlands

It was noticed that hyperestrogenia is a widespread syndrome in female allergic rhinitis (AR) sufferers. The main evidence of this syndrome in a female organism are mastopathy and pre-menstrual syndrome (PMS). Long-term administration of OC leads to an increased level of hyperestrogenia as well. We have interrogated 500 women suffering from AR and perennial rhinitis (PR). It was revealed that only 20% of patients do not have those symptoms. Eighty percent suffer from either one or both.

We investigated the occurrence of ER-β in the tissue of patients suffering from nasal polyp (NP), because a biopsy from an AR patient is not allowed. The aim of this investigation is the localization of ER-ß in nasal mucosa.

The tissue (mucosa of inferior turbinate and polyp tissue) of 30 patients who underwent surgical treatment was the object of the study. Polyp tissue and turbinate tissue of 20 patients suffering from NP (ten female and ten male patients) were obtained with a FEES procedure. The control group was nasal mucosa from the inferior turbinate of ten patients (five female and five male patients) suffering from a deviation of the septum nasi without allergy in anamnesis. The average age of the examined patients was 35 years. Nasal turbinates, mucosa and polyp tissue were used for immunohistochemical studies.

Immunohistochemical analysis of the tissue clearly showed the presence of ER-β-positive cells, which were situated particularly in the epithelial cells and interstitial space. ER-β-positive cells were found in the tissue of the lower turbinate as well as in the tissue of the polyp. Differences between the quantity of ER-β, dependent on the sex of the patients, were not detected. Analyzing the received data, it is important to point out that ER-β-positive cells that are situated in the glands were detected only in the tissue of the polyps.

These results affirm the presence of ER-β in the lower turbinate tissue and polyp tissue, and the quantity does not depend on the sex of the patient.

Taking into account the fact that in patients with AR and NP high levels of estrogen were found, we conducted an experiment, where we investigated the influence of tamoxifen (drugs with anti-estrogen properties and stimulation β-receptors) on the development of AR (unfortunately, we do not have an experimental animal model of NP).

Table 1. The influence of Tamoxifen on the nasal mucosa in the experiment

Measure	Control (n=20)	Allergic rhinitis (n=20)	Allergic rhinitis and tamoxifen treatment (n=20)
Quantity of masteocytes	16±0.9	43±2.3	33±1.3
Coefficient of degranulation	107.5±2.4	291.1±2.4	222±3.0
Measure of profile field	0.3±0.004	0.89±0.005	0.59±0.002

Tamoxifen inhibits the development of allergic reactions in the nasal cavity, which is manifested in the reduction of the number of mastocytes, coefficients of degranulation and magnitudes of profile fields (table 1).

The results may enable the development of a new treatment approach of NP and AR by medical agents that stimulate the action of ER-β.

This has been successfully done in other areas of medicine.

COMPLEMENTARY AND ALTERNATIVE THERAPY OF RHINOSINUSITIS

G.C. Passali[1], L.M. Bellussi[2], F.M. Passali[3], D. Lucidi[1], D. Passali[2]

[1]*Department of ENT, Catholic University of the Sacred Heart, Rome, Italy;*
[2]*Department of ENT, University of Siena, Italy;* [3]*Department of ENT, Tor Vergata University, Rome, Italy*

According to the International Rhinosinusitis Advisory Board,[1] goals of rhinosinusitis therapy are: to treat the infection, to shorten the disease and to prevent the recurrences. In order to achieve these goals, many different pharmacological approaches have been tested by several study groups. Acute rhinosinusitis (ARS) resolves without antibiotic treatment in most cases, symptomatic treatment and reassurance is the preferred initial management strategy for patients with mild symptoms. Antibiotic therapy should be reserved for patients with severe ARS, especially in presence of high fever or severe (unilateral) facial pain. Clinicians should weigh the moderate benefits of antibiotic treatment against the potential for adverse effects.

The aim of a pharmacological approach in ARS is represented by the opening of the ostia while in chronic inflammatory processes of the nose and paranasal sinuses, the goal is rather to restore a healthy respiratory mucosa.[2] Corticosteroids, local decongestants, non-steroidal anti-inflammatory drugs (NSAD) antihistamines, mucolytic agents, SPA therapy are considered adjunctive therapies in acute and chronic rhinosinusitis both in adults and children. Local decongestants are useful in treating nasal obstruction and ostia blockage thus preventing complications, although they are characterized by notable side effects (such as rebound and tachyphylaxis), reasons why the use of this therapy is not recommended for a period longer than seven to ten days. Topical steroids, such as Fluticasone Furoate, Mometasone Furoate, or Budesonide are widely-used medicaments, in association to antibiotics, both in acute and chronic pathology of the nose and sinuses. In acute rhinosinusitis they have shown a significant

Address for correspondence: Dr. Giulio Cesare Passali, Department of Head and Neck Surgery, Institute of Otorhinolaryngology, Catholic University of the Sacred Heart, Largo A. Gemelli 8, 00168, Rome, Italy. Tel: +390630154439. Fax:+39063051194. E-mail: giulio.passali@rm.unicatt.it

Recent Advances in Rhinosinusitis and Nasal Polyposis, pp. 33-38
Edited by Hideyuki Kawauchi, Desiderio Passali, Ranko Mladina, Andrey Lopatin
and Dmytro Zabolotnyi
2015 © Kugler Publications, Amsterdam, The Netherlands

improvement in nasal subjective symptoms (such as nasal secretions, cough, congestion, facial pain), although no radiological evidence of mucosal thickening and inflammation decrease was proven.[3-4] On the contrary, both subjective and objective (hystopathological, radiological and functional) advantages have been demonstrated by the association of topical steroids and antibiotics in the management of chronic rhinosinusitis (CRS) by many studies.[5] In particular, a significant decrease in major basic protein (MBP)-positive eosinophils and tryptase-positive mast cells in the epithelium and lamina propria was shown in patients affected by perennial rhinitis who underwent a 12-months treatment period with mometasone furoate aqueous nasal spray, in absence of adverse tissue changes.[6]

The *European Position Paper on Rhinosinusitis and Nasal Polyps* (EP3OS) 2012 pointed out the clinical irrelevance of mucolytic agents in acute disease, while the use of antihistamines seems appropriate in allergic population only.[2] Administration of antimicrobial therapy, especially in CRS, may not be regardless of the existence of bacterial biofilm. A wide variety of otolaryngologic diseases, such as chronic otitis media, chronic adeno-tonsillitis, cholesteatoma as well as chronic rhinosinusitis, have been associated to development of self-assembling bacterial surface-attached communities representing an ancient prokaryotic survival strategy: in mucosal biofilm, in fact, different set of genes expressed by bacteria, particular communication and signaling pathways, alternative mechanisms to diffuse nutrients, compared with planktonic bacteria, are responsible for antimicrobial resistance and protection from host defense.[7] An interesting paper in a pediatric subset of patients explains as bacterial biofilm in the nasopharynx of children with CRS may act as a chronic reservoir for bacterial pathogens, resistant to standard antibiotics.[8] Current therapeutic strategies are aimed at inhibition of biofilm aggregation, biofilm disruption and pathogens eradication. It is proven that subclinical doses of macrolides inhibit signaling within and between bacterial communities[9] while N-acetyl-cysteine (NAC) seems to break up biofilm network in a dose-dependent way.[10]

Historical use of saline nasal irrigation, douches, sprays and rinsing is maintained, as an adjunct to the medical management of both chronic and acute inflammatory disease of the nose and paranasal sinuses. Nasal saline lavages decrease the contact time between irritants, infective agents or pollutants and nasal mucosa. Two different Cochrane reviews analyze the available evidences on nasal washing in chronic and acute rhinosinusitis and their efficacy towards comparative treatments. It has been demonstrated that, in ARS, saline nasal irrigation is helpful in reducing nasal symptom score and objective nasal patency, both alone and in combination to antibiotics and topic decongestants.[11] In the management of CRS, a review by Harvey and co-workers[12] has confirmed that saline is beneficial in the treatment of chronic symptoms, both as the only treatment modality and as adjunct therapy; hypertonic solution is suggested to be more effective by selective researches although unsurprisingly saline irrigation in not as effective as topical steroids. A Japanese study by Kim and colleagues[13] compared the effects of hypo-, iso-, and hypertonic saline irrigation on mucus secretion and cellular morphology in cells cultures, and demonstrated that isotonic saline treatment (0,9%) is the most physiologic treatment in terms of both items, while hypotonic (0,3%) and hypertonic (3%) saline irrigations may produce various degrees of cellular damage, (such as ciliary rupture and number decrease, exfoliation of secretory cells or mucin active secretion). *In-vivo* studies[14] recommend the use of nasal rinsing with hypertonic solution in a pediatric population affected by seasonal allergic rhinoconjunctivitis, as it was proven to reduce the mean weekly rhinoconjunctivitis score and intake of oral antihistamines in absence of adverse effects.

Inhalation of thermal water is not included among the management options by the most recent guidelines, although it represents a traditional tool in chronic sinonasal diseases and chronic bronchitis. A guideline recently published by the Italian Society of Otorhinolaryngology[15] evidences the lack of correct indications of SPA therapy in relation to different chemical and physical characteristics of spring water, whereas its efficacy is nowadays documented by several subjective and objective parameters. Spring waters are classified according to physical and chemical features (temperature, pressure, ionic concentration, radioactivity, presence of specific ions or active chemical groups). Their mechanism of action is mechanical (cleansing, massage), immunological (through the activation of macrophages and immunoglobulins production) and neuro-vegetative (through the stimulation of hypothalamus-hypophysis axis and autonomic innervation). A recent study[16] highlighted the active role of SPA therapy with radioactive hydrofluoric oligominerals waters in chronic inflammation of the upper airways. Specifically, a reduction of neutrophilic infiltration at the rhinocytogram and the improvement of the mucociliary function, recorded as muco-ciliary transport time (MCTt) values, was proven. Sulphurous water has beneficial effects on mucus secretions.[17] Because of the slight toxicity of sulphide groups, this water has antimicrobial effects, immunomodulant activity (increase of blood and nasal secretory IgA), together with decrease of mucus viscosity.[18] Glycosaminoglycans (GAGs) are heterogeneous polysaccharides which fill the extracellular matrix of the respiratory system. Their function is to regulate hydration and water homeostasis, to maintain structure and function and to modulate the inflammatory response and tissue remodelling.[19] A paper by Soldati et al.[20] underlined the role of hyaluronic acid-containing cream in mucosal wound healing after nasal surgery, showing a decrease in the presence of crusts and improvement in respiration. It also produces a subjective relief as it is judged useful by the patient especially in limiting the presence of local lesions and blood clots. Hyaluronic acid represents a useful tool also in the management of the 'empty nose syndrome', *i.e.* the nasal atrophy secondary to extensive nasal surgery.[21] Results from a recent *in-vitro* study suggest that retinoid acid, released from supportive biomaterial, persists locally for almost seven days and induces mucociliary and aquaporin expression and differentiation.[22] This statement may lead to future therapeutic applications in postoperative mucosal restoration.

An increasing body of evidence is, at present, available regarding the use of phytotherapy or probiotics but a more systematic review on their efficacy and safety profile is needed.

Increase in allergy prevalence in the last decades is attributed to changes in exposure to microbial stimulus in childhood; this theory provides a rational for the use of probiotics in primary prevention in order to modify the gut microbial environment and modulate the immune response.[23] Moreover, probiotics might also be tested for secondary treatment in allergic patients basing on immune modulation theory, especially in children.

Complementary-Alternative Medicine (CAM) is frequently employed in treatment of allergic diseases, including asthma and rhinitis, but evidence-based recommendations are lacking, moreover, methodology of related clinical trials results often inadequate.[24]

No clear evidence is offered for the efficacy of acupuncture and physical techniques (breathing control, yoga, chiropractic manipulation) in the treatment of allergic-asthmatic patients, although some papers report the increase of subjective satisfaction and quality of life scores. Some positive results were described in rhinitis treated with homeopathy in good quality trials[25] but a small number of negative reports counterbalance this data.

Regarding phytotherapy, the use of raw extracts from natural origin as medicines, there are some studies that report positive results of drugs derived from plants and herbs (such as Boswellia Serrata, Tylophora indica, grapeseed and butterbur extracts) in the treatment of asthma, bronchoconstriction and rhinitis.[26-27] More structured investigations are required for extracts standardization and analysis of side effects and interactions.

Modern technologies allow optimization of the extracts in order to enhance their effects: using sophisticated separation technologies, partial extracts are produced which contain the particularly effective ingredients in higher concentrations compared to the original extract.

Phytoneering stands for the decipherment of the major potential of plants (phytos) with the use of the most modern research and innovative technologies (engineering), to produce effective and safe herbal products.

The dry extract BNO1011 (Sinupret® Bionorica SE) is based on a combination of five herbs and is used to treat acute and chronic rhinosinusitis: in experimental *in-vitro* and *in-vivo* researches, as well as in clinical studies, this extract has shown anti-inflammatory,[28] antiviral[29] activities and mucolytic/mocokinetic effects through stimulation of transepithelial chloride transport.[30]

In conclusion, considering that topical corticosteroids, local decongestants, non-steroidal anti-inflammatory drugs (NSAD), antihistamines and mucolytic agents are regularly included in standard therapeutic protocols for acute and chronic inflammation of the nose and paranasal sinuses, in our opinion probiotics, SPA therapy, nasal lavages and phytoteraphy may be considered, basing on the evidences offered in this review and also on the evidence obtained in the patient's treatment, not as complementary therapy but as crucial as 'regular' therapy in the management of rhinosinusitis.

References

1. International Rhinosinusitis Advisory Board. Infectious rhinosinusitis in adults: classification, etiology and management. Ear Nose Throat J 1997;76(12 Suppl):1-22.
2. Fokkens WJ. et al. EPOS 2012: European position paper on rhinosinusitis and nasal polyps 2012. A summary for otorhinolaryngologists .Rhinology 2012;50(1):1-12.
3. Meltzer EO, Charous BL, Busse WW,et al. Added relief in the treatment of acute recurrent sinusitis with adjunctive mometasone furoate nasal spray. The Nasonex Sinusitis Group. J Allergy Clin Immunol 2000;106(4):630-637.
4. Nayak AS, Settipane GA, Pedinoff A, et al.; Nasonex Sinusitis Group. Effective dose range of mometasone furoate nasal spray in the treatment of acute rhinosinusitis. Ann Allergy Asthma Immunol 2002;89(3):271-278.
5. Lund VJ1, Black JH, Szabó LZ, Schrewelius C, Akerlund A. Efficacy and tolerability of budesonide aqueous nasal spray in chronic rhinosinusitis patients. Rhinology 2004;42(2):57-62.
6. Minshall E1, Ghaffar O, Cameron L, et al. Assessment by nasal biopsy of long-term use of mometasone furoate aqueous nasal spray (Nasonex) in the treatment of perennial rhinitis. Otolaryngol Head Neck Surg 1998;118(5):648-654.
7. Post JC, Stoodley P, Hall-Stoodley L, Ehrlich GD. The role of biofilms in otolaryngologic infections. Curr Opin Otolaryngol Head Neck Surg 2004;12(3):185-190.
8. Coticchia J, Zuliani G, Coleman C, et al. Biofilm surface area in the pediatric nasopharynx: Chronic rhinosinusitis vs obstructive sleep apnea. Arch Otolaryngol Head Neck Surg 2007;133(2):110-114.
9. Swords WE, Rubin BK. Macrolide antibiotics, bacterial populations and inflammatory airway disease. Neth J Med 2003;61(7):242-248.
10. Bozzolasco M., Debbia EA., Schito GC. GIMMOC 2002;6(3):203-215.
11. Kassel JC, King D, Spurling GK. Saline nasal irrigation for acute upper respiratory tract infections. Cochrane Database Syst Rev 2010;(3):CD006821.
12. Harvey R, Hannan SA, Badia L, Scadding G. Nasal saline irrigations for the symptoms of chronic rhinosinusitis. Cochrane Database Syst Rev 2007;18:(3):CD006394.
13. Kim CH, Hyun Song M, Eun Ahn Y, Lee JG, Yoon JH. Effect of hypo-, iso- and hypertonic saline irrigation on secretory mucins and morphology of cultured human nasal epithelial cells. Acta Otolaryngol 2005;125(12):1296-1300.
14. Garavello W, Di Berardino F, Romagnoli M, Sambataro G, Gaini RM. Nasal rinsing with hypertonic solution: an adjunctive treatment for pediatric seasonal allergic rhinoconjunctivitis. Int Arch Allergy Immunol 2005;137(4):310-314.
15. Linee Guida relative alla procedure terapeutiche termali attinenti la specialità di Otorinolaringoiatria. Argomenti di Acta Otorhinolaryngologica Italica. Vol. I. N. 1 Maggio 2007.
16. Passali D, De Corso E, Platzgummer S, et al. Spa therapy of upper respiratory tract inflammations. Eur Arch Otorhinolaryngol 2013;270(2):565-570.
17. Salami A, Dellepiane M, Crippa B, et al. Sulphurous water inhalations in the prophylaxis of recurrent upper respiratory tract infections. Int J Pediatr Otorhinolaryngol 2008;72(11):1717-1722.
18. Staffieri A, Abramo A. Sulphurous-arsenical-ferruginous (thermal) water inhalations reduce nasal respiratory resistance and improve mucociliary clearance in patients with chronic sinonasal disease: preliminary outcomes. Acta Otolaryngol 2007;127(6):613-617.
19. Souza-Fernandes AB, Pelosi P, Rocco PR. Bench-to-bedside review: the role of glycosaminoglycans in respiratory disease. Crit Care 2006;10(6):237.

20. Soldati D, Rahm F, Pasche P. Mucosal wound healing after nasal surgery. A controlled clinical trial on the efficacy of hyaluronic acid containing cream. Drugs Exp Clin Res 1999;25(6):253-261.
21. Modrzyński M. Hyaluronic acid gel in the treatment of empty nose syndrome. Am J Rhinol Allergy 2011;25(2):103-106.
22. Huang TW, Chan YH, Su HW, Chou YS, Young TH. Increased mucociliary differentiation and aquaporins formation of respiratory epithelial cells on retinoic acid-loaded hyaluronan-derivative membranes. Acta Biomater 2013;9(6):6783-6789.
23. Kalliomäki M, Antoine JM, Herz U, et al. Guidance for substantiating the evidence for beneficial effects of probiotics: prevention and management of allergic diseases by probiotics. J Nutr 2010;140(3):713S-721S.
24. Passalacqua G, Bousquet PJ, Carlsen KH, et al. ARIA update: I--Systematic review of complementary and alternative medicine for rhinitis and asthma. J Allergy Clin Immunol 2006;117(5):1054-1062.
25. Reilly DT, Taylor MA, McSharry C, Aitchison T. Is homoeopathy a placebo response? Controlled trial of homoeopathic potency, with pollen in hayfever as model. Lancet 1986;2(8512):881-886.
26. Gupta I, Gupta V, Parihar A, Gupta S, Lüdtke R, Safayhi H, Ammon HP. Effects of Boswellia serrata gum resin in patients with bronchial asthma: results of a double-blind, placebo-controlled, 6-week clinical study. Eur J Med Res 1998;3(11):511-514.
27. Schapowal A; Petasites Study Group. Randomised controlled trial of butterbur and cetirizine for treating seasonal allergic rhinitis. BMJ 2002;324(7330):144-146.
28. Rossi A, Dehm F, Kiesselbsch C, et al. The novel Sinupret® dry extract exhibits anti-inflammatory effectiveness in vivo. Fitoterapia 2012;83:715-720.
29. Glatthaar-Saalmuller B, Rauchhaus U, Rode S, Haunschild J, Saalmuller A. Antiviral activity in vitro of two preparations of the herbal medicinal product Sinupret® against viruses causing respiratory infections. Phytomedicine 2011;19:1-7.
30. Kreindler JL, Chen B, Kreitman Y, et al. The novel dry extract BNO 1011 stimulates chloride transport and ciliary beat frequency in human respiratory epithelial cultures. Am J Rhinol Allergy 2012; 26(6):439-443.

ANTROCHOANAL POLYPS VERSUS NASAL POLYPS

Ranko Mladina

ORL Department, Clinical Hospital Center Zagreb, Zagreb, Croatia

When speaking of antrochoanal polyps and nasal polyposis in general, one has to bear in mind that the use of endoscopes made possible to finally get very deep and close to the real roots of the nasal polyps which gives rise to the hope that one day it will be possible to eradicate nasal polyps surgically for once and for all, *i.e.*, without the need of repeated surgical interventions, long-term use of the steroid drugs, etc. On the other side, one has to bear in mind the fact that so-called accessory ostia of the maxillary sinus do not exist at all, *i.e.*, that only one natural ostium of the maxillary sinus exists in reality. Therefore, all other 'holes' that can be seen at the lateral nasal wall during endoscopy mean the same: the defect of the lateral nasal wall tissue as a consequence of spontaneous disruption of some neglected empyema of the maxillary sinus and because of that a chronic inflammation of the maxillary sinus itself. Furthermore, it seems that the cyst at the posterior wall of the maxillary sinus in cases of antrochoanal polyps (ACP) is not just a simple retention cyst as other cysts in this sinus are. It rather is a circumscribed inflammation of the regional mucosa of grade 2 to 3 after Terrier's classification.

In cases of antrochoanal polyps, one part of this formation (a cystic one) is located within the maxillary sinus, more precisely (and absolutely unexpectedly for the cystic formation within the maxillary sinus), it is attached at its posterior wall, and then, through the defect of the lateral nasal wall (not at all through the natural ostium!) it comes out into the nose and forms a 'hanging polyp' formation that apparently belongs to the ostiomeatal complex as nasal polyps usually do, but this one is always solitary, absolutely never truss-like, that is: it is the only one, single polyp! So, when operating an antrochoanal polyp it is not enough to remove the 'polypous' part from the nasal cavity and then get into the maxillary sinus and pull out the cyst. What one has to perform is to

Address for correspondence: Prof. Dr. Ranko Mladina, 10.000 Zagreb, Hrastik 11 A, Croatia. E-mail: rmladina@gmail.com

Recent Advances in Rhinosinusitis and Nasal Polyposis, pp. 39-40
Edited by Hideyuki Kawauchi, Desiderio Passali, Ranko Mladina, Andrey Lopatin and Dmytro Zabolotnyi
2015 © Kugler Publications, Amsterdam, The Netherlands

precisely identify the natural ostium first, and then to 'unify' the natural ostium and the defect of the posterior fontanellae so as to connect them, *i.e.*, to make a widely open approach to the posterior sinus wall.

As to the recurrences of nasal polyps, one should think of the possible role of the biofilm. Biofilm is a complex, organized aggregation of bacteria in an extracellular matrix which is adhered to an underlying surface. It is detectible by different methods: *in vitro*, through different microscopy techniques (scanning electron microscopy (SEM), transmission electron microscopy (TEM), confocal laser microscopy) and detection of genes with biofilm-forming capacity. Recent publications estimate that at least 65% of all human bacterial infections involve biofilms. Bacteria anchored in biofilm are protected from their external environment by the density of the matrix. On the other hand, low level of metabolic activity of bacterial cells makes them almost immune to the effects of antibiotics. These facts support persistence and survival of bacteria in biofilms for long periods of time. So far, biofilms have been associated with a number of chronic diseases, such as chronic otitis media, chronic adenoiditis, endocarditis, dental plaque, etc. Chronic rhinosinusitis and nasal polyposis are new objectives in the studies on biofilms. It has recently been shown that biofilms are present on the removed tissue of 80% of patients undergoing surgery for chronic sinusitis. A study on mucosal changes in CRS revealed different degrees of denudation (loss of cilia and goblet cells), resulting in a surface prone to biofilm formation. Another study showed a correlation between the marked biofilm-forming capacity by *Pseudomonas aeruginosa* and *Staphylococcus aureus* on one side and the persistence of chronic sinusitis and nasal polyposis following ESS on the other.

As to the recurrence of ACP, it must be pointed out that the wall of the sinus cyst histologically shows very loose, edematous stroma full of inflammatory cells and dilated vessels, suggesting chronic inflammation. According to Kern and Zinreich, chronic osteomyelitis can be found in almost all cases of chronic sinusitis. Inflammation of the bone produces the sequestration. A new, avascular bone replaces sequestered parts forming so-called involcrum (meaning an envelope), containing exudates and debris, therefore supporting the maintenance of the chronic inflammation. In addition, recent molecular studies of the ACP showed up-regulation of bFGF (basic fibroblast growth factor), up-regulation of TGF (transforming growth factor) and up-regulation of MUC genes (MUC 5AC, MUC 5B, MUC 8), thus suggesting the importance of the local inflammatory reaction. Thus, the surgery for antrochoanal polyps performed in this way diminishes the chances for recurrences, which at the moment, even in cases operated endoscopically, seems to range between three up to 16%.

COMPLICATIONS OF FUNCTIONAL ENDONASAL SINUS SURGERY

D. Passali, J. Cambi, L. Bellussi

ENT Department, University of Siena, Siena, Italy

Introduction

In 1929, Mosher wrote that endonasal ethmoid surgery was the most danger-ous of all surgical operations.[1] This is why the extra-nasal approach has been preferred by surgeons and viewed as associated with less risk of complications.

In the 1970s, advances in endoscopes and operating microscopes, as well as improved understanding of the conformation and pathophysiology of the paranasal sinuses played a major role in the renaissance of functional endonasal sinus surgery (FESS).[2]

Minor and major complications can be distinguished in endonasal ethmoid surgery:[3] some may occur during the operation, others in the post-operative period, others in both. Minor complications have an incidence of about 3% and are associated with modest morbidity, whereas major complications only have an incidence of about 0.5% but are associated with significant morbidity, often require urgent treatment and may have very bad outcome for patients (Table 1).

Complications may even occur when the surgeon has extensive experience in nasal surgery; however, there are three distinct phases in the sinus surgery learning curve:

1. Phase I (1-30 operations): greatest risk of complications, mostly with dural injury.
2. Phase II (30-100 operations): lower risk of complication, mostly with peri-orbital injuries.
3. Phase III (> 100 operations): lowest risk, mostly rare but serious complica-tions.[4]

Address for correspondence: Desiderio Passali MD PhD, ENT Department, Università di Siena, Viale Bracci, 11 53100, Siena, Italy. E-mail: d.passali@virgilio.it

Recent Advances in Rhinosinusitis and Nasal Polyposis, pp. 41-51
Edited by Hideyuki Kawauchi, Desiderio Passali, Ranko Mladina, Andrey Lopatin and Dmytro Zabolotnyi
2015 © Kugler Publications, Amsterdam, The Netherlands

Table 1. Major and minor complications.

	Major	Minor
Intra-operative	Periorbital emphysema Bleeding Optic nerve lesion Medial rectus damage Retro-orbital haemorrhage CSF leakage	Bleeding Fat herniation Nasolacrimal duct
Post-operative	Bleeding CSF leakage	Synechiae Epiphora Periorbital emphysema Diplopia Olfactory impairment Atrophic rhinitis Neuropathic pain Bleeding

Concerning the possible severity of complications, sinus surgery remains one of the most dangerous fields of surgery in otorhinolaryngology. A good nose surgeon should be able to prevent and master every complication that can arise from surgical procedures. This chapter will focus on selected complications of endonasal sinus surgery.

Minor complications

Epiphora

The nasolacrimal duct may be damaged during antrostomy, since if the latter extends too far anteriorly it damages the lacrimal sac or nasolacrimal duct. The best way to avoid damage is not to extend the ostium anteriorly. If the duct is damaged, epiphora is generally transitory and the duct recanalizes into the nose, making treatment unnecessary. Epiphora can be prolonged if scarring, stenosis or infection of the duct occurs. In the case of osteitis or infection, there may be dacrocystitis and purulent discharge from the medial corner of the affected eye. Persistent cases may require ophthalmological assessment by nasolacrimal duct probing or stenting, with severe cases requiring dacrocystorhinostomy. Antibiotic-steroid eye cream and/or oral antibiotics are needed in patients with evidence of infection. Warm compresses, nasal saline spray and decongestants can help.[5,6]

Periorbital emphysema

If the lamina papyracea is interrupted, and the patient has blown his/her nose in the first four days or choked a sneeze, this can force air into the soft tissues in the region of the eye. This may be further aggravated if the patient sneezes, coughs, cries or lifts weights. Periorbital swelling and crackling can be detected during assessment. Ecchymosis may accompany the emphysema.

If the lamina papyracea defect is recognized during the operation, the anaesthetist must be instructed not to press too much if the patient requires ventilation with a facemask. If emphysema occurs, it will resorb provided the patient does not blow any more air into the area. Prophylactic antibiotics are prescribed to avoid periorbital cellulites.[7]

Diplopia

Diplopia can be determined by injury to the ocular medial rectus and superior oblique muscles. Because it passes lateral to the periorbita towards the middle of the lamina papyracea, the injury mainly involves the medial rectus muscle. The medial rectus muscle is less protected by the layer of fat posteriorly and damage results in strabismus and disturbing diplopia. The injury can be caused by direct cutting of the muscle or its nearby vascular and nerve supply. Spontaneous healing seldom occurs. Permanent diplopia is a very rare complication that requires neuro-ophthalmological assessment and possibly strabismus surgery.[8,9]

Synechiae

The most common postoperative complication of FESS is synechiae, which occur in 6-22% of cases, even with adequate local homecare. They most frequently occur between the middle turbinate and the lateral nasal wall. If the surgeon removes too much and manipulates the region of the frontal recess, synechiae leading to frontal rhinosinusitis may arise. Occlusion of the surgical antrostomy or osteomeatal complex may predispose to recurrent maxillary infections.

Prevention is by fine dissection and cutting tissue towards diseased regions, avoiding mucosal scratching and tearing. Mitomycin-C has also been applied to diminish the incidence of scarring, ostium closure and synechiae.[10] Placing Merocel® or a silicone stent between the middle turbinate and lateral nasal wall may facilitate healing while avoiding scarring of the middle turbinate and lateralization. Very close postoperative follow-up until re-epithelisation is the most successful way of preventing synechiae. Around 15% of patients with synechiae need second surgery.[11]

Olfactory impairment

Olfactory mucosa extends from the cribriform plate to the entire medial face of the middle turbinate. To avoid injury to the olfactory mucosa, it helps to administer preoperative oral steroids, especially if polyps are medial to the middle turbinate according to preoperative endoscopy. If polyps are mainly medial to the middle turbinate, during surgery it is best to perform a complete ethmoidectomy and then softly lateralize the middle turbinate to open up the olfactory area. If the anterior end of the middle turbinate adheres to the lateral wall, complete ethmoidectomy aerates the maxillary sinus. The technique decreases the risk of adhesions in this area and permits better access to nasal steroids. If a patient has hyposmia after FESS and the middle turbinate adheres to the septum, it can help to resect these and lateralize the middle turbinate as an elective procedure after any mucosal oedema has subsided.[12]

Atrophic rhinitis

When the mucosa is damaged, cilial mucus secretion may take months to return to physiological levels. In this case, the following may help: regular douching, hydration, vapour inhalation (not too hot) and humidifying ambient air. In a minority of patients, areas of mucosa can become dry and atrophic. Various ointments have been used to prevent drying out. Radiotherapy patients and those with ciliary dyskinesia will need to wash and hydrate the nose indefinitely.

Neuropathic pain

Trauma or surgery causes pain mediated by myelinated A delta and unmyelinated C fibres. Prolonged stimulation can turn on N-methyl-D-aspartate (NMDA) receptors and cause central sensitization. In a small percentage of patients, central processing can lead to hyperalgesia, or spontaneous firing of neurons due to modification in pain thresholds. These patients are rarely helped by nonsteroidal anti-inflammatory drugs. They often respond to amitriptyline, carbamazepine or gabapentin.[13] The treatment of postsurgical pain should be primarily with neuroactive pharmacological agents, which are helpful in many patients.

Frontal recess stenosis

Often the frontal recess and frontal sinus accumulate mucus that is released once the nasal cavity is freed of polyps. It is therefore important not to attack this region without significant reason.

The take-home message is not to deprive the frontal recess of its mucosa, as this may cause stenosis. The best thing to do if there is a purulent disease in the frontal sinus is to open the frontal recess using a 45° endoscope, dissect the mucosa off the agger nasi air cells with a ball probe and then pull the probe down onto the shell of the cell and remove the bone fragments. If you cannot find the recess, it is best not to push the probe in a random way because CSF leaks, orbital damage or frontal stenosis are often determined by non-standard manoeuvres. In the case of revision of frontal recess stenosis, computer-aided surgery can be used.[14]

Major complications

Bleeding

Bleeding is inevitable during surgery and can be minimized by maximizing preoperative medical management with corticosteroids and antibiotics and re- moving tissue with through-cutting forceps or a shaver to avoid tearing the mucosa. Anaesthetic management is important to reduce intraoperative bleeding. Anaesthesia with high remifentanil and low blood pressure is preferred. Before starting surgery, 20° body-up, arterial mean pressure between 65 and 75 mmHg, decongestion with topical vasoconstrictors on nasal pledgets, followed by good infiltration with 1% lidocaine with epinephrine are essential. Waiting less than seven to ten minutes after the injection is a frequent error. The other main causes of bleeding, besides clotting disorders, are related to the sphenopalatine artery and the anterior ethmoid artery.

Major vessel injury and brain haemorrhage

Injury to major blood vessels, like the internal carotid artery, and brain are extremely rare during FESS. Injury to the internal carotid artery is much more common during sphenoid sinus surgery. In 20% of sphenoid sinuses the bony carotid canal may be dehiscent. Before opening the sphenoid sinus, the surgeon must review the axial CT to consider a protruding internal carotid artery. If it is possible to visualise the natural opening of the sphenoid sinus, this can be ex- panded. The anterior wall of the sphenoid sinus is removed by working medially with downbiting and upbiting forceps. It is important to be very watchful with surgical manipulations at the intersphenoidal septum. The septum sphenoidalium may be anchored posteriorly to a thin carotid artery canal and should not be fractured but removed solely with cutting instruments or a diamond drill. This manoeuvre can lead to partial laceration of the carotid artery and development of a false aneurysm, sometimes weeks or even months later.[15]

In the case of injury to the carotid artery, surgery must be suspended im- mediately and the sphenoid sinus filled with haemostatic material. Even if the bleeding seems under control, it is necessary to watch for development of a false aneurysm. If this does not occur, the sinus is best repacked with fascia and fat followed by oxidized cellulose, and a pack is left in place for a week. If bleed- ing continues when the pack is gently removed, the radiologist should be asked to do an occlusion study under EEG control. If there are no EEG changes after occlusion or the patient is instable, it is best to close the artery by endovascular coiling or by a transcranial approach with the help of a neurosurgeon.

Sphenopalatine artery

The artery may bleed during FESS in the following cases:

- If the middle meatal antrostomy is opened posteriorly to less than 0.5 cm from the posterior wall of the maxillary antrum;
- If a branch comes through the inferior turbinate;
- If another branch comes through the middle turbinate and bleeds when more than half of the anterior part of the middle turbinate is removed;
- If the sphenoid ostium is opened below halfway up its height, the posterior tributary of the sphenopalatine artery will be open.

Cauterization with bipolar diathermy is usually sufficient to stop the bleeding.

Anterior ethmoid artery

Cutting the anterior ethmoid artery can have severe consequences. When the artery retracts into the orbit, it can cause a sharp increase in posterior compartment pressure. This condition will prejudice the vessels of the optic nerve and retina, leading to blindness. The surgeon should not operate if he cannot see anything. If bleeding is not controlled somehow it is better to abort the operation than to cause damage. Most complications during FESS take place in the final part of the operation, when the surgeon removes small residual polyps, which in itself is of little benefit.

The anterior ethmoid artery is seldom responsible for postoperative bleeding but if so, it can be diathermied.

CSF leakage

The surgeon causes a CSF leakage when he accidentally perforates the skull base. This happens most frequently at:

- The anterior ethmoid roof in the region of the lateral lamella of the cribriform plate;
- The junction between the posterior ethmoid roof and the sphenoidal plane.

If the olfactory furrow is deep in relation to the ethmoid roof (type III according to Keros)[16] there might only be a very thin bony border dividing the olfactory groove from the ethmoidal cavity. To avoid damage, the cribriform plate is a useful reference for the anterior half of the middle turbinate when performing dissection in the ethmoid region. The surgeon should always stay lateral to the middle turbinate, because medial dissection may lead to a CSF fistula. CSF leaks documented intraoperatively must be stopped immediately to avoid risk of meningitis. The long-term results of intraoperative duraplasty are excellent.[17]

Postoperative CT is highly recommended to assess any possible intracranial injury, and this may require collaboration with the neurosurgeon. A skull-base defect resulting from endonasal sinus surgery can almost always be closed using an endonasal approach.

To avoid CSF leakage we suggest:

- Avoiding tinkering where the middle turbinate attaches to the roof of the anterior skull base;
- Finding the height of the roof of the sphenoid sinus and then opening the posterior ethmoid air cells;
- Not angling surgical instruments medially toward the lateral lamella of the cribriform plate;
- Flexing the head on the neck, so that the skull base lies in a more vertical plane;
- Studying the CT: a 'black halo' of air in the peripheral cells around the skull base is an encouraging sign, whereas a CT 'white-out' calls for a more prudent approach.

Orbital complications

Lamina papyracea

Damage to the lamina papyracea can determine ecchymosis and periorbital emphysema. Periorbital emphysema typically arises when some air enters the soft tissues surrounding the orbit, typically when the patient awakes coughing or if blowing the nose. Crackling of soft tissue, a soft bulb and no decrease in vision are typical signs of emphysema. Management is simple observation and educating patients not to blow their nose. Emphysema usually reabsorbs within seven to ten days.[18]

In revision FESS and massive polyposis, the risk of injury to the lamina papyracea increases because it may be reduced or partially dehiscent. Limited damage to the lamina papyracea is not a serious complication. In cases of laceration of the periorbita, periorbital fat typically bulges out and can be recognized by its yellow colour.

The bulb-pressing test, as described by Draf and Stankiewicz, can be helpful when there is no doubt about injury of the lamina papyracea and/or periorbita. Herniated fat should not be removed. If a small fat herniation is noted, no treatment is necessary. If a large fat herniation occurs, gentle replacement is indicated and sealing with connective tissue transplants. Postoperative antibiotic treatment is recommended in these circumstances. The axis of the pupils should be evaluated to check for any medial rectus damage or grade of proptosis. In such situations, urgent ophthalmological assessment is required.

Orbital haematoma

Orbital haematoma mainly occurs after penetration of the lamina papyracea. The veins that run along the lamina papyracea are more likely to determine orbital haematoma than damage to the ethmoid arteries.[19] Although rare, laceration of one of the ethmoid arteries is a severe complication. The vessel may retract into the orbit, leading quickly to retrobulbar haematoma. It is advisable to avoid working at the edge of the orbit if the course of the artery is not clear. If the artery is damaged at this point, it immediately retracts just inside the orbit and cannot be cauterized.

Untreated orbital haematoma determines an increase in orbital pressure and proptosis, which may lead to temporary visual impairment or blindness[20] caused by reduced vascular supply to the optic nerve, which is very susceptible to ischaemia. In this case, immediately reduce intraorbital pressure by removing nasal packing, raising the head, medical treatment (antihypertensives, diuretics and corticosteroids) and surgical treatment. Surgical treatment in these circumstances is lateral canthotomy followed by inferior cantholysis and possibly superior cantholysis, which provide immediate orbital decompression.[21] In addition, transnasal orbital decompression by removing the lamina papyracea and incision of the orbital periosteum may also be considered.

Medial rectus damage

Medial rectus damage is due to inattention: if the orbital periosteum is crossed, the assisting surgeon should observe movement of the eye. Damage to the medial rectus normally occurs through deeper penetration into the orbit. Unfortunately, even if it is recognized at the time, it is very difficult to avoid the scarring and diplopia that are likely to occur. Even expert strabismus surgeons have difficulty improving problems caused by damage to the medial rectus.

Optic nerve trauma

The optic nerve can be damaged by penetration of the orbit through the lamina papyracea but the surgeon may not realize he has entered the orbit. Direct damage to the optic nerve is less common than indirect injury via retrobulbar haematoma. Typical high-risk areas are the sphenoid sinus and posterior ethmoid, especially when there is extensive pneumatisation.[22] In these situations, it is first advisable to find the sphenoid sinus medially and then work forward. The optic nerve can be prominent in 20% of patients in the upper half of the lateral wall of the sphenoid sinus, but it is rarely dehiscent. Fortunately, direct optic nerve injury is extremely rare and only a few individual cases have been described.[23]

Incidence and our experience

Major complications are estimated to arise in one to three percent of patients, based on early studies with relatively small patient cohorts in academic institutions. Synechiae and intra-operative bleeding are the first and second most frequent complication, respectively, in all reports. Orbital complication and CSF leakage are the most serious complications. Table 2 shows the incidence rates recorded by several sinus surgeons.

Table 2. Incidence rates in major sinus surgery international departments.

Surgeon [ref] N patients Complication	Castillo [24] 553	Jakobsen [25] 237	May [26] 2108	Danielsen [27] 230	Rudert [28] 1172	Stankiewicz [29] 3402	Ramakrishnan [30] 62823
Orbital haematoma	0.18%	0%	0.05%	0%	0.25%	/	/
CSF leakage	0.18%	0,54%	0.5%	0%	0.8%	0.55%	0.17%
IO bleeding	0.36%	21%	0.9%	4.34%	0.8%	1.20%	0.76%
PO bleeding	1.08%	0%	0%	0%	0%		
Lacrimal duct lesion	0.36%	/	0%	0%	0%	/	/
Synechiae	3.07%	20%	6.9%	6.52%	/	/	/
Lamina papyracea	2%	0%	0%	2.6%	0%	/	/
Diplopia	0%	/	0%	0%	/	/	/
Orbital lesion	/	0%	0%	0%	0%	0.85%	0.07%
Olfactory impairment	/	/	/	/	/	/	/

In the period January 1980 to June 2014, 3504 adult patients underwent FESS in our Department. Intra-operative bleeding complicated 3.2% of operations. Post-operative bleeding occurred in 4.8%. The major risk factors for bleeding were revision surgery and hypertension. There were no significant differences in the incidence of complications between males/females and different age groups. In our experience, major complications are very rare. Orbital haematoma complicated 0.05% of FESS. We did not record any cases of diplopia or CSF leakage after FESS, probably because of optimal pre-operative anaesthesiological and radiological assessment. Our surgeons also have long training targeted at avoiding surgical aggression by preserving anatomical landmarks. After primary surgery, it is therefore always possible to make minor retouches under local anaesthesia, for example for synechiae or small localized recurrence of polyps.

Table 3 shows the incidence rates recorded in our Department.

Table 3. Incidence rates in the Siena ENT Department.

	3480 paz
Orbital haematoma	(5) 0.14%
CSF leak	0
IO bleeding	(111) 3.2%
PO bleeding	(167) 4.8%
Lacrimal duct lesion	0
Synechiae	N.R.
Lamina papyracea	(35) 1%
Diplopia	0%
Orbital lesion	0%
Olfaction impairment	/

References

1. Mosher H. The surgical anatomy of the ethmoid labyrinth. Ann Otol Rhinol Laryngol 1929;38:869-901.
2. Draf W. Endoscopy of the Paranasal Sinuses. Berlin/Heidelberg/New York: Springer 1983.
3. May M, Levine HL, Schaitkin B, et al. Complications of endoscopic sinus surgery. In: Levine HL, May M (Eds.), Endoscopic Sinus Surgery, pp 193-124. New York: Thieme 1993.
4. Keerl R, Stankiewicz J, Weber R, Hosemann W, Draf W. Surgical experience and complications during endonasal sinus surgery. Laryngoscope 1999;109:546-550.
5. Cohen NA, Antunes MB, Morgenstern KE. Prevention and management of lacrimal duct injury. Otolaryngol Clin North Am 2010;43:781-788.
6. Bolger WE, Parsons DS, Mair EA, Kuhn FA. Lacrimal drainage system injury in functional endoscopic sinus surgery. Incidence, analysis, and prevention. Arch Otolaryngol Head Neck Surg 1992;118:1179-1184.
7. Rodriguez MJ, Dave SP, Astor FC. Periorbital emphysema as a complication of functional endoscopic sinus surgery. Ear Nose Throat J 2009;88:888-889.
8. Dutton JJ. Orbital complications of paranasal sinus surgery. Ophthalmic Plast Reconstr Surg 1986;2:119-127.
9. Thacker NM, Velez FG, Demer JL, Wang MB, Rosenbaum AL. Extraocular muscle damage associated with endoscopic sinus surgery: an ophthalmology perspective. Am J Rhinol 2005;19:400-405.
10. Numthavaj P, Tanjararak K, Roongpuvapaht B, McEvoy M, Attia J, Thakkinstian A. Efficacy of Mitomycin C for postoperative endoscopic sinus surgery: a systematic review and meta-analysis. Clin Otolaryngol 2013;38:198-207.
11. Stammberger H, Posawetz W. Functional endoscopic sinus surgery. Concept, indications and results of the Messerklinger technique. Eur Arch Otorhinolaryngol 1990;247:63-76.
12. Pade J, Hummel T. Olfactory function following nasal surgery. Laryngoscope 2008;118:1260-1264.
13. Yin HL, Chui C, Tung WF, Chen WH. Nummular headache after trans-sphenoidal surgery: a referred pain-based headache syndrome. Neurol Neurochir Pol 2013;47:398-401.
14. Rombaux P, Ledeghen S, Hamoir M, et al. Computer assisted surgery and endoscopic endonasal approach in 32 procedures. Acta Otorhinolaryngol Belg 2003;57:131-137.
15. Lister JR, Syper GW. Traumatic false aneurysm and carotid-cavernous fistula: a complication of sphenoidotomy. Neurosurgery 1979;5:473-475.
16. Keros P. Über die praktische Bedeutung der Niveauunterschiede der Lamina cribrosa des Ethmoids. Z Laryngol Rhinol 1965;41:808-838.
17. Schick B, Weber R, Mosler P, Keerl R, Draf W. Long-term follow-up of fronto-basal duraplasty. HNO 1997;45:117-122.

18. Stankiewicz JA. Complications of endoscopic sinus surgery. Otolaryngol Clin North Am 1989;22:749-758.
19. Stankiewicz JA, Chow JM. Two faces of orbital hematoma in intranasal (endoscopic) sinus surgery. Otolaryngol Head Neck Surg 1999;120:841-847.
20. Oeken J, Bootz F. Severe complications after endonasal nasal sinus surgery. An unresolved problem. HNO 2004;52:549-553.
21. Saussez S, Choufani G, Brutus JP, Cordonnier M, Hassid S. Lateral canthotomy: a simple and safe procedure for orbital haemorrhage secondary to endoscopic sinus surgery. Rhinology 1998;36:37-39.
22. Hosemann WG, Weber RK, Keerl RE, Lund VJ. Minimally Invasive Endonasal Sinus Surgery. Stuttgart/New York: Thieme 2000.
23. Kim JY, Kim HJ, Kim CH, Lee JG, Yoon JH. Optic nerve injury secondary to endoscopic sinus surgery: an analysis of three cases. Yonsei Med J 2005;46:300-304.24. Castillo L, Verschuur HP, Poissonnet G, Vaille G, Santini J. Complications of endoscopically guided sinus surgery. Rhinology 1996;34:215-218.
25. Jakobsen J, Svendstrup F. Functional endoscopic sinus surgery in chronic sinusitis – a series of 237 consecutively operated patients. Acta Otolaryngol Suppl 2000;543:158-161.
26. May M, Levine HL, Mester SJ, Schaitkin B. Complications of endoscopic sinus surgery: analysis of 2108 patients – incidence and prevention. Laryngoscope 1994;104:1080-1083.
27. Danielsen A, Olofsson J. Endoscopic endonasal sinus surgery. A long-term follow-up study. Acta Otolaryngol 1996;116:611-619.
28. Rudert H, Maune S, Mahnke CG. Complications of endonasal surgery of the paranasal sinuses. Incidence and strategies for prevention. Laryngorhinootologie 1997;76:200-215.
29. Stankiewicz JA, Lal D, Connor M, Welch K. Complications in endoscopic sinus surgery for chronic rhinosinusitis: a 25-year experience. Laryngoscope 2011;121:2684-2701.
30. Ramakrishnan VR, Kingdom TT, Nayak JV, Hwang PH, Orlandi RR. Nationwide incidence of major complications in endoscopic sinus surgery. Int Forum Allergy Rhinol 2012;2:34-39.

SINUS CRISTAE GALLI – CONSTANTLY NEGLECTED SOURCE OF CHRONIC INFLAMMATION OF PARANASAL SINUSES

R. Mladina

Clinical Hospital Center Zagreb, Zagreb, Croatia

Because the crista is part of the ethmoid bone and the ethmoid complexes are pneumatized at birth, it seems reasonable that some crista galli pneumatization would be present if the pneumatizing cells were from the ethmoid complex. But, crista galli is never ossified at that time, it is still cartilaginous. Most ossification of the cartilaginous crista galli starts at approximately two months of postnatal life, steadily increases in ossification to 14 months of age, and then slowly progresses until it finishes by 24 months of age. According to Dodd, Jing[1] and Netter[2], the development of the frontal bone is much slower. Frontal sinuses do not reach the level of the superior orbital rims before six to seven years of age. The question arises here why we cannot find any pneumatization of the crista galli in children younger than seven years of age? The explanation came a few years ago from Som and his group[3], who proved that the pneumatization of the crista galli comes from the frontal sinus itself, not from the ethmoid. They also found that the frequency of pneumatizations increases with age, *i.e.*, it was not observed in the kindergarten group (0-7 yrs of age), but its frequency raised to 4% in the elementary school age (7-14) whereas it was seen in 14% of the patients older than 14 yrs of age. No data of sex differences were mentioned in their report.

Pneumatization of the crista galli can easily be recognized on CT scans, but unfortunately it is usually neglected not only by radiologists, but also by rhinologists all over the world. Our experience, however, has proven this anatomical entity to be even more frequent than Som *et al.*[3] found in their material: we found it at CT scans of 37.5% of our CRS patients. The minimal anterio-posterior dimension was 5.1 millimeter, and latero-lateral 7.1 millimeter. After observing a huge number of patients having a pneumatized crista galli, we found out that

Address for correspondence: Prof. Dr. Ranko Mladina, 10.000 Zagreb, Hrastik 11 A, Croatia.
E-mail: rmladina@gmail.com

Recent Advances in Rhinosinusitis and Nasal Polyposis, pp. 53-54
Edited by Hideyuki Kawauchi, Desiderio Passali, Ranko Mladina, Andrey Lopatin
and Dmytro Zabolotnyi
2015 © Kugler Publications, Amsterdam, The Netherlands

this entity has remarkable influence on the clinical picture, particularly in cases of chronic rhinosinusitis followed by frontal headache, hyposmia or even anosmia!

Several cases of chronic inflammation and other pathological entities of the pneumatized crista galli are presented. It is high time to start calling this anatomical entity by the name it deserves: 'sinus cristae galli'.

References

1. Dodd G, Jing B. Radiology of the Nose, Paranasal Sinuses, and Nasopharynx. Baltimore: Williams & Wilkins;1977 :60
2. Netter F. Atlas of Human Anatomy. Summit, NJ: Ciba-Geigy;1989 :44
3. Som PM, Park EE, Naidich TP, Lawson W. Crista galli pneumatization is an extension oft he adjacent frontal sinuses. Am J Neuroradiol 2009; 30: 31-33

THE ROLE OF MACROLIDES IN QUALITY OF LIFE IN NASAL POLYPS PATIENTS MANAGED WITH OPTIMAL MEDICAL THERAPY

B.S. Gendeh[1], S.K. Aboud[2], S. Husain[1]

[1]Department of Otorhinolaryngology, Universiti Kebangsaan Malaysia, Jalan Yaacob Latif, Cheras, Kuala Lumpur, Malaysia; [2]Department of Otorhinolaryngology – Head and Neck Surgery, Malaysian Allied Health Sciences Academy (MAHSA) University, Jalan Elmu off Jalan Universiti, Kuala Lumpur, Malaysia

Abstract

Background: Nasal polyps (NP) have an enormous impact on quality-of-life (QOL) and its management involves a combination of medical and surgery therapy. Macrolides constitutes the mainstay of conservative therapy in NP, both in primary treatment and to prevent recurrence. To the authors' knowledge, no publication has extensively examined NP after optimal medical treatment based on subjective evaluations. The aims of this prospective study were designed to evaluate the QOL in NP patients after: (1) initial three-months course of macrolide; (2) a short course of oral steroids; (3) long-term treatment with intranasal steroids.

Methods: Fifty-five patients with grade I and II NP were consecutively treated with macrolide 250 mg daily for the first three months, single-dose oral prednisolone 25 mg for two weeks (medical polypectomy), and long-term intranasal steroids. Patients were followed-up and evaluated at base line, three, six, and 12 months for QOL measure.

Results: At baseline, patients with grade I and grade II NP showed significantly worse QOL scores on all Rhinosinusitis Disability Index (RSDI) domains, mainly for physical function (4.59 ± 1.41) and predominantly higher in social function (3.16 ± 1.17). At three, six, and 12 months of treatment, patients demonstrated

Address for correspondence: Dr. Balwant Singh Gendeh, MS (ORL-HNS), Department of Otorhinolaryngology, Universiti Kebangsaan Malaysia, Jalan Yaacob Latif, 56000 Cheras, Kuala Lumpur, Malaysia. E-mail: bsgendeh@gmail.com

Recent Advances in Rhinosinusitis and Nasal Polyposis, pp. 55-62
Edited by Hideyuki Kawauchi, Desiderio Passali, Ranko Mladina, Andrey Lopatin and Dmytro Zabolotnyi
2015 © Kugler Publications, Amsterdam, The Netherlands

a significant improvement in all impaired QOL domains compared to baseline after optimal medical therapy ($p < 0.05$).

Conclusion: These results suggest that the optimal medical treatment to improve QOL incorporates medical polypectomy with macrolide and maintained by long-term intranasal steroid therapy. Our findings demonstrate that clarithromycin has a strong anti-inflammatory effect on NP patients.

Introduction

Nasal polyps (NP) are characterized by a recurrent sinonasal mucosal inflammatory process with the presence of two or more symptoms that include obstruction, congestion or discharge, facial pain or pressure and reduced sense of smell for more than 12 weeks. Of late, there has been increasing interest in the immunomodulatory actions of macrolides, mainly in chronic rhinosinusitis and NP. Numerous studies have been conducted by Japanese and other investigators on the efficiency of long-term, low-dose therapy with 14-membered ring macrolides for the treatment of chronic rhinosinusitis and NP. NP formation and growth are activated and perpetuated by an integrated process involving the mucosal epithelium, lamina propria and inflammatory cells, which may be initiated by both infectious and non-infectious inflammation.[1] Inflammatory mediators such as IL-1B,IL-5,IL-6,IL-8 and RENTES are present in nasal polyps.[2-4] Various toxic agents, infectious agents and allergens, encountered at the level of the nasal and paranasal mucosa may activate innate immune mechanisms and lead to induction of pro-inflammatory cytokines. Reduction in the size of the NP could be a result of two associated processes: suppression of NP fibroblast proliferation and chemokine production in NP fibroblasts. The decrease in size of NP correlates significantly with the reduction in the concentration of IL-8 in nasal lavage from these patients.[3]

There is lack of documentation in prospective, randomized, controlled trials regarding improvement of QOL after medical treatment of NP which suggest that surgical treatment of NP has a better effect on QOL than medical treatment.[5] QOL improvement after NP treatment is correlated to nasal symptom scores. The most commonly used validated questionnaires to assess QOL are the RSDI which utilizes three subscales (emotional, physical and functional) to aggregate measurements of general health status and disease-specific QOL.[6] Nasal endoscopy has a prominent role in detecting NP, primarily a disease managed by optimal medical therapy pre- and post-surgery.[7] Macrolide antibiotics have high anti-inflammatory activity and decrease the virulence of colonizing bacteria which leads to shrinkage of NP by suppressing cytokine production by inflammatory cells in the paranasal sinus epithelium.[8]The main aims of this study were: (1) to evaluate the QOL outcomes in patients with grade-I and grade-II NP after optimal medical therapy; (2) to evaluate the frequency of various diseases in NP patient; (3) to correlate nasal symptoms score and QOL after medical therapy.

Materials and methods

Study population

Fifty-five patients with NP grades I and II (Lildholdt classification) were included in this prospective evaluation from April 2011 to February 2013 with age range of 18 to 65 years with mean age of 51.47 (standard deviation (SD) ± 14.35). Females outnumbered males (54.5% and 45.5%). Study approval was obtained from the Ethics Committee and a signed informed consent was obtained. All patients were examined, treated and followed-up by the same rhinologist for the entire duration of the study at the outpatient Otorhinolaryngology clinic. The diagnosis of NP was based on the documented medical history and on the results of clinical examination and nasal endoscopy (using rigid optic 0 and 30 degree endoscope; Storz, Tuttlingen, Germany).

Inclusion and exclusion criteria

The inclusion criteria were patients with age 18-65 years, nasal symptoms more than 12 weeks and NP grades I and II. The exclusion criteria were NP grade III, surgically treated patient with NP, pregnancy, macrolide hypersensitivity, patients with absolute contraindications for systemic steroids, liver or gastrointestinal dysfunction and with severe structural abnormalities caused by deviated nasal septum.

Study design

Fifty-five patients received macrolide antibiotic 250 mg daily for the first three months, a 25-mg dose of systemic steroid (oral prednisone) once daily for two weeks, followed by a long-term intranasal steroid (*e.g.*, mometasone furoate aqueous nasal spray 200 mcg/day). Initial baseline evaluation before treatment was performed followed by three follow-up evaluations at three, six and 12 months of treatment. Nasal symptoms and QOL were scored by RSDI questionnaire and all the recruited patients underwent skin-prick test.

Nasal symptoms score

Rhinorrhea, sneezing, nasal obstruction and loss of smell were recorded. The severity of these symptoms was assessed and scored on subsequent follow-up: 0, excellent; 1 and 2, very good; 3 and 4, good; 5 and 6 fair; 7 and 8, poor; 9 and 10, very poor.

QOL and Rhinosinusitis Disability Index assessment

All patients with grade-I and -II NP fulfilling the inclusion criteria were assessed subjectively pre- and post-medical treatment by the RSDI questionnaire

(28 questions) divided into three domains (physical, mental and social). Scale scores range from 0 to 100% and lower scores indicate better QOL. Each domain has ten levels of answers based on tables which permit only one answer and scores were noted and compared at different follow-up study interval (baseline, three, six and 12 months).

Statistical analysis

Data analysis was performed with the statistical package IBM SPSS version 19.0 using mean ± SD. A *P*-value of < 0.05 was considered statistically significant. All data was assessed for normal distribution. A paired t-test was used to compare the score of mean over time. QOL (physical, mental and social) and treatment were compared to baseline scores by two-tailed paired Student's t-test and differences between groups were assessed using the t-test. The chi-square test was used to look for associations (numbers and percentages) among the group. ANOVA was used to compare 55 patients' percentages of QOL and nasal symptoms scores for different time visit.

Results

Fifty-five NP patients were prospectively recruited and enrolled into the study with baseline comparison of disease-severity scores (*i.e.*, QOL scores) and a one-year follow-up. All patients received medical co-interventions (oral clarithromycin, prednisolone, and continuous intranasal steroid) and allergy therapy. Follow-up data was available for 55 (91%) of the 60 patients at the completion of the study.

Frequency of various diseases in nasal polyps

Prior to treatment, twenty patients of NP were diagnosed as hypertensive (36.4%). Allergic rhinitis, asthma, eczema, and aspirin intolerance were seen in 17 (30.9%), 19 (34.5%), 5 (9.1%) and 3 (5.5%) NP patients respectively. Amongst 55 patients with nasal polyposis only 39 (70.9%) were under medication (Table 1).

Nasal symptoms scores

Patients scored loss of smell and nasal obstruction as major complaints. At three, six and 12 months all nasal symptoms significantly improved compared to baseline. However, loss of sense of smell worsened at 12 compared to six months. At baseline, asthmatic patients with NP had higher scores of nasal obstruction (6.68 ± 1.38) and loss of sense of smell (6.68 ± 1.80) than non-asthmatics (5.78 ± 1.84 and 6.17 ± 1.95 respectively)($P < 0.05$). At three and six months, asthmatic and non-asthmatic patients scored similar improvement in nasal obstruction and loss of sense of smell.

Table 1. Disease condition by duration visit (N = 55).

	Baseline		3 Months		6 Months		1 Year	
Disease	N	%	N	%	N	%	N	%
DM	12	21.8	9	16.4	7	12.7	8	14.5
HT	20	36.4	18	32.7	17	30.9	17	30.9
Asthma	19	34.5	16	29.1	15	27.3	16	29.1
AR	17	30.9	16	29.1	14	25.5	15	27.3
Osteoporosis	1	1.8	1	1.8	1	1.8	1	1.8
Aspirin intolerance	3	5.5	3	5.5	3	5.5	3	5.5
Eczema	5	9.1	5	9.1	5	9.1	5	9.1
Hypothyroidism	2	3.6	2	3.6	2	3.6	2	3.6

Quality of life (RSDI) assessment

ANOVA was used to compare 55 patients' percentages of QOL for various duration visits. Pair-wise comparisons showed the QOL baseline (40.52 ± 12.07) was significant at three months (23.66 ± 9.85), six months (18.32 ± 8.42) and one year (17.28 ± 8.79) follow-up (Table 2). In comparison of percentages of QOL by time of visit, patients with NP had significantly worse QOL scores before treatment. At three months, patients with NP showed a similar significant improvement in QOL. In all domains of RSDI, patients with NP showed significantly worse physical function (4.59 ± 1.41) QOL scores than social function (3.16 ± 1.17). All the RSDI domains are statistically correlated to NP patients with asthma (Table 3). At baseline, asthmatic patients with NP had worse scores of QOL ($P < 0.05$) than non-asthmatic patients with NP in physical, mental and social functioning.

Discussion

The population characteristics were similar to the literature with reference to age (mean = 51 years), sex ratio (1.19), prevalence of associated asthma (34.5%), and sensitivity to aspirin (5.5%).[9-11] Our study highlighted that (1) both clarithromycin and steroid treatments maintain improvement in nasal symptoms; (2) patients with NP have a significantly worse QOL in all RSDI domains (physical functioning lower than mental). Our study reveals that QOL in patients with NP is impaired where physical health is more impaired than the mental, and a short course of oral steroids caused a significant improvement in all domains of RSDI; long-term treatment with clarithromycin and intranasal steroids maintained this improvement. The two most disabling symptoms in baseline NP patients were reduced sense of smell and nasal obstruction. Short-term systemic steroid administration thus appears to have the same efficacy as polypectomy, but the

Table 2. Comparison of mean percentages QOL by duration visit.

		Mean	Std. deviation	Paired t-test	P
Pair 1	**QOL baseline**	40.52	12.07		
	QOL 3 months	23.66	9.85	18.22	0.001*
	QOL 6 months	18.32	8.42	18.66	0.001*
	QOL 12 months	17.28	8.79	19.30	0.001*

* Significant P < 0.05

Table 3. Comparison of mean physical, mental and social components in asthmatic and non-asthmatic patients with NP.

	Physical		
	All (N = 55)	*No asthma (N = 33)*	*Asthma (N = 19)*
T0	4.59 ± 1.41	4.48 ± 1.43	4.79 ± 1.37
T3	2.80 ± 1.27*	2.65 ± 1.23*	3.09 ± 1.32*
T6	2.21 ± 0.99*	2.18 ± 1.08*	2.27 ± 0.82*
T12	2.03 ± 1.05*	2.04 ± 1.17*	2.02 ± 0.81*

	Mental		
	All (N = 55)	*No asthma (N = 33)*	*Asthma (N = 19)*
T0	3.70 ± 1.19	3.58 ± 1.10	3.92 ± 1.34
T3	2.07 ± 0.83*	2.00 ± 0.89*	2.20 ± 0.69*
T6	1.59 ± 0.81*	1.56 ±0 .86*	1.65 ± 0.73*
T12	1.49 ± 0.95*	1.50 ± 1.01*	1.48 ± 0.86*

	Social		
	All (N = 55)	*No asthma (N = 33)*	*Asthma (N = 19)*
T0	3.16 ± 1.17	3.05 ± 1.15	3.36 ± 1.22
T3	1.65 ± 0.81*	1.60 ± 0.85*	1.77 ± 0.75*
T6	1.53 ± 1.42*	1.33 ± 0.73*	1.91 ± 2.19*
T12	1.24 ± 0.77*	1.21 ± 0.69*	1.30 ± 0.91*

T0, Baseline; T1, 3 Months; T2, 6 Months; T3, 1 Year, *Paired t-test with baseline, **P < 0.001**.

improvement proves to be short-lived.[12] Topical therapy has a definite beneficial effect on the clinical disorders and on the polyp size, but shows little activity on the sense of smell dysfunction.

A study of 20 patients with CRS and NP treated for a minimum of three months with clarithromycin 400 mg/d revealed that in the group whose polyps were reduced in size, the IL-8 levels decreased fivefold. The IL-8 levels were also significantly higher before macrolide treatment than in the group whose polyps showed no change.[13] IL-8 may be related to nasal polyp shrinkage due to macrolide suppression of cytokine production in inflammatory cells in sinus epithelium.[14,15]

In another uncontrolled trial, 40 patients were treated with roxithromycin 150 mg for eight weeks; the lower-grade NP shrunk in about half of the patients and no correlation was found between treatment effect and extent of eosinophilia in the tissue.[16] Macrolides effectively decreased the size of the NP despite the presence of allergies or the extent of eosinophilic infiltration. Macrolides have both direct inhibitory effects on epithelial secretory cells and indirect anti-inflammatory effects resulting in polyp shrinkage. Moreover, they reduce the concentrations of pro-inflammatory cytokines, reduce neutrophil migration and inflammatory mediators and inhibit the proliferation of fibroblasts that are important in pathogenesis of chronic sinusitis.[17-19] An in-vitro study showed that macrolides reduce proliferation of fibroblasts in NP.[20] The clinical benefit of macrolides includes decreased nasal secretion and postnasal drip with improvement in nasal obstruction.

Literature revealed a greater impairment of QOL when NP was associated with asthma and physical and mental functioning were significantly lower in asthmatics than in non-asthmatics. Asthma had an adverse impact on vitality and general health compared with rhinosinusitis, but no significant differences in postoperative SF-36 scores from patients with rhinosinusitis.[21] This study revealed that asthmatic patients had a higher nasal symptom score and worse QOL for physical, mental and social functioning than non-asthmatics. However, asthmatic and non-asthmatics had similar nasal symptoms, polyp size, and scored similar QOL domains after oral steroids, and these effects were maintained by long-term intranasal steroid therapy.

In conclusion, the strength of this study includes sample size, length of follow-up, the prospective nature of data collection and rigorous methodology used to qualify QOL. The main limitation is that it was a subjective evaluation of QOL by RSDI questionnaire leading to biasness. A very small sample of patients with aspirin intolerance resulted in biasness when compared to 52 patients with aspirin tolerance.

References

1. Norlander T, Bronnegard M, Stierna P. The relationship of nasal polyps, infection and inflammation. Am J Rhinol 1999;13:349-355.
2. Bachet C, Wagenmann M, Rudack C, et al. The role of cytokines in infectious sinusitis and nasal polyposis. Allergy 1998;53:2-13.
3. Allen JS, Eisma R, LaFreniere D, et al. Interleukin-8 expression in human nasal polyps. Otolaryngol Head Neck Surgery 1997;117:535-541.
4. Bachet C, Wagenmann M, Hauser u, Rudack C. IL-5 synthesis is upregulated in human nasal polyp tissue. J Allergy Clin Immunol 1997;99:837-842.
5. Ragab SM, Lund, VJ, Scadding G. Impact of chronic rhinosinusitis therapy on quality of life; A prospective randomized controlled trial. Rhinology 2010;48:305-311.

6.   Benninger MS, Senior, BA. The development of Rhinosinusitis Disability Index. Arch Oto-
     laryngol Head Neck Surg 1997;123:1175-1179.
7.   Shahizon AMM, Suraya A, Rozman Z, et al. Correlation of computed tomography and nasal
     endoscopic findings in chronic rhinosinusitis. Med J Malaysia 2008;63:211-215.
8.   Katsuta S, Osafune H, Takita R. Therapeutic effect of roxithromycin on chronic sinusitis
     with nasal-polyps, clinical, computed tomography and electron microscopy analysis. Nihon
     Jibiinkoka Gakkai Kaiho 2002;105:1189-1197. [In Japanese.]
9.   Brown BL, Harner SG, van Dellen RG. Nasal polypectomy in patients with asthma and
     sensitivity to aspirin. Arch Otolaryngol 1979;105:413-416.
10. Drake-Lee AB, Lowe D, Swanston A, et al. Clinical profile and recurrence of nasal polyps.
     J Laryngol Otol 1984;98:783-793.
11. Larsen K, Tos M. The estimated incidence of symptomatic nasal polyps. Acta Otolaryngol
     2002;122:179-182.
12. Lildholdt T, Mygind N. Effect of corticosteroids on nasal polyps: evidence from controlled
     trials. In: Mygind N, Lildholdt T (Eds.), Nasal polyposis: An Inflammatory Disease and Its
     Treatment, pp. 160-169. Copenhagen: Munksgaard 1997.
13. Yamada T, Fujieda S, Mori S, et al. Macrolide treatment decreased the size of nasal polyps
     and IL-8 levels in nasal lavage. Am J Rhinol 2000;14:143-148.
14. Ichimura K, Shimazaki Y, Ishibashi T, Higo R. Effect of new macrolide roxithromycin upon
     nasal polyps associated with chronic rhinosinusitis. Auris Nasus Larynx 1996;23:48-56.
15. Nonaka M, Pawankar R, Tomiyama S, et al. A macrolide antibiotic, roxithromycin, inhibits
     the growth of nasal polyp fibroblasts. Am J Rhinol 1999;13:267-272.
16. Wallwork B, Coman W, Feron F, Mackay-Sim A, Cervin A. Clarithromycin and prednisolone
     inhibit cytokine production in chronic rhinosinusitis. Laryngoscope 2002;112:1827-1830.
17. Suzuki H, Shimomaru A, Ikeda K, et al. Inhibitory effect of macrolides on interleukin-8
     secretion from cultured human nasal epithelium cells. Laryngoscope 1997;107:1661-1666.
18. Nonaka M, Pawankar R, Saji F, Yagi T. Effect of roxithromycin on IL-8 synthesis and
     proliferation of nasal polyp fobroblasts. Acta Otolaryngol Suppl. 1998;539:71-75
19. Nonaka M, Pawankar R, Tomiyama S, Yagi T. A macrolide antibiotic, roxithromycin inhibits
     the growth of nasal polyp fibroblasts. Am J Rhninol 1999;13:267-272.
20. Winstead W, Barnett S. Impact of endoscopic sinus surgery on global health perception: an
     outcomes study. Otolaryngol Head Neck Surg 1998;119:486-491.
21. Alobid I, Benítez P, Bernal-Sprekelsen M. Nasal polyposis and its impact on quality of life.
     Comparison between the effects of medical and surgical treatments. Allergy 2005;60:452-
     458.

THE ROLE OF ENDOSCOPIC SURGERY IN SINONASAL PAPILLOMAS

B.S. Gendeh[1], S.K. Aboud[2], S. Husain[1]

1Department of Otorhinolaryngology, Universiti Kebangsaan Malaysia, Jalan Yaacob Latif, Kuala Lumpur, Malaysia; ²Department of Otorhinolaryngology – Head and Neck Surgery, Malaysian Allied Health Sciences Academy (MAHSA) University, Jalan Elmu off Jalan Universiti, Kuala Lumpur, Malaysia

Introduction

Papillomas of the nasal cavity may be classified in 3 distinct categories: inverted, fungiform, and cylindrical. Fungiform papillomas arise from the nasal septum, whereas inverted and cylindrical papillomas typically arise from the lateral nasal wall. Although benign in nature, they can extend beyond their site of origin and destroy bone and recur when incompletely excised. Malignant degeneration can occur in 5-20% of inverted papillomas. They are most commonly diagnosed in white males during the fifth to the seventh decade (mean 50 years).Complete resection has been the criterion standard for the treatment of these lesions. Traditionally, a lateral rhinotomy with a medial maxillectomy were recommended; however, endoscopic approaches have slowly become the standard treatment. One challenge for the planning of its surgical excision is that the lesion tends to be more extensive than clinical examination suggest. In addition, 12-30% of inverted papillomas are multicentric.[1] Excision with negative margins may be difficult and incomplete removal invariably leads to recurrence. In most series using traditional approaches, the recurrence rate is 10-30%.

Inverted papilloma are benign sinonasal tumors that have a propensity to recur after surgical resection and may undergo malignant transformation. Therefore, a complete resection is essential for the successful management of these tumors. Advances in Endoscopic techniques and experience as well as improved radiologic accuracy and navigation are increasing the role of minimally invasive, endoscopic approaches for surgical resection of inverted papilloma.

Address for correspondence: Dr Balwant Singh Gendeh, MS (ORL-HNS), Department of Otorhinolaryngology, Universiti Kebangsaan Malaysia, Jalan Yaacob Latif, 56000-Cheras, Kuala Lumpur, Malaysia. E-mail: bsgendeh@gmail.com

Recent Advances in Rhinosinusitis and Nasal Polyposis, pp. 63-66
Edited by Hideyuki Kawauchi, Desiderio Passali, Ranko Mladina, Andrey Lopatin and Dmytro Zabolotnyi
2015 © Kugler Publications, Amsterdam, The Netherlands

Materials and methods

There are no published data on the prevalence of HPV in inverted papilloma in Malaysia. HPV prevalence rates in inverted papillomas vary widely. A meta-analysis by Lawson showed prevalence of HPV in IP ranged between 0-76.9percent.[2] A cross sectional study done showed one of 29 patients (3%) with Inverted Papilloma was positive for HPV. A total number of 44 paraffin-embedded tissue (PET) samples between Jan 2001 till October 2013 were collected. All past and newly diagnosed samples were retrieved from the Department of Pathology archive of Universiti Kebangsaan Malaysia Medical Centre (UKMMC). Specific PET blocks containing tissues with IP were identified and chosen for sectioning and PCR analysis. The statistical software SPSS (SPSS, Inc., Chicago, USA, PASW Statistics for Windows, version 20) was used to analyse the differences in the frequency of HPV genotypes from the cases with sinonasal inverted papillomas. HPV status and genotypes were analysed with clinico-pathological variables using the Chi square test (2-tailed) or Fisher's exact test (2- tailed) where applicable.

Majority of the patients underwent endoscopic modified medial maxillectomy, frontal sinustomy, ethmoidectomy, wide maxillary antrostomy and sphenoidotomy.

Result

Forty four patients with sinonasal papillomas attending the Otorhinolaryngology Clinic of UKMMC from January 2001 to October 2013 were included in the study. There were 36 males and 8 female patients(5;1).The mean age of the males was 60 years(18-72) and females was 56 years(41-68).

The most prevalent type of HPV detected in the samples was Type 11 which was detected in eight (18%) patients. There were five (11%) patients that were positive for HPV Type 6. Four patients had HPV Type 16 (9%) while only two (5%) patients had HPV type 18 detected. Eleven out of 34 (32%) patients with IP had at least one positive HPV detected. Two out of seven (29%) patients with tumour recurrence had at least one type of HPV positivity. Two out of three (67%) patients with IP with SCC had at least one type of HPV detected. Four patients were found to have two subtypes present from the histological specimens. One of the patients had Type 6 and Type 11 HPV, another patient had Type 6 and Type 16 present while two more patients had type 16 and Type 18 HPV detected (Table 1). None of the patients had more than two subtypes present. The most prevalent type of HPV detected in the samples was Type 11 which was detected in eight (18%) patients. There were five (11%) patients that were positive for HPV Type 6. Four patients had HPV Type 16 (9%) while only two (5%) patients had HPV type 18 detected. Eleven out of 34 (32%) patients with IP had at least one positive HPV detected. Two out of seven (29%) patients with tumour recurrence had at least one type of HPV positivity. Two out of three (67%) patients with IP with SCC had at least one type of HPV detected.

Table 1. Number of patients with low risk and high risk HPV detection according to histological features

	Total Number of Patients	HPV 6&11 (Low Risk)	HPV 16 & 18 (High Risk)	HPV 6 & 16
IP	34	–	–	1
IP with recurrence	7	1	–	–
IP with SCC	3	–	2	–
Total	44	1	2	1

Discussion

Refinements in endoscopic techniques have led to a paradigm shift for the resection of inverted papilloma. Endoscopic resection offers the advantage of avoiding incisions and in most patients can be performed as ambulatory surgery. The extent of the procedure is customized accordingly to the extent of the disease, including total ethmoidectomies, wide maxillary antrostomies, sphenoidotomies, frontal recess exploration, and turbinate resection, if required. Once all visible papillomas are removed, any residual tumors are eliminated by drilling over its site of origin. In experienced hands, endoscopic resection has a recurrence rate that is equal to that of traditional techniques.[3, 4] Outcomes using endoscopic techniques compare favorably with that of open approaches. Long-term endoscopic surveillance and frequent follow-up are crucial, regardless of the surgical technique. Recurrence is usually discovered 12-20 months after surgery but has been reported as late as 30-56 months.[3] In selected cases, endoscopic management is a useful approach with favorable outcomes and less morbidity when compared with more aggressive surgical approaches.[5] Recent advances in preoperative imaging, intraoperative navigation system, endoscopic instrumentation, and hemostatic materials have made endoscopic resection of nasal and paranasal sinus tumors a viable alternative to the traditional techniques. Its role in resecting small lesions confined to the nasal cavity is well established. With increasing experience, endoscopic endonasal approaches have expanded beyond the nasal cavity and paranasal sinuses to areas such as the infratemporal fossa and cranial cavity. Endoscopic techniques can be used alone or in combination with open approaches, according to the different degree of involvement of the anterior skull base Advantages of the endoscopic approach include the avoidance of facial incisions, low morbidity and shorter length of hospital stay. Early oncologic outcomes are at least equivalent to those of open approaches, however, long long-term follow-up and larger cohorts of patients are needed before it gains universal acceptance.[6, 7]

Contraindications to a completely endoscopic endonasal approach include invasion of the orbit, involvement of superficial tissues such as the anterior and lateral portion of the frontal sinus, anterior wall of the maxillary sinus and nasal bones, and invasion of the skin.

Conclusion

The prevalence of HPV detected in inverted papillomas in our patients is 34% which supports the theory that HPV infection plays an aetiological factor in sinonasal inverted papilloma. Moreover, a high dectection rate of high risk HPV type(67%) was observed in patients with inverted papilloma with malignant transformation. Furthermore, this supports the theory that high risk HPV plays a role in the oncogenesis of sinonasal inverted papilloma. Thus, this study implicates that HPV sub-type testing may identify patients at high risk for recurrence, or progression to dysplasia and malignancy.

Advances in Endoscopic techniques and experience as well as improved radiologic accuracy and navigation are increasing the role of minimally invasive, endoscopic approaches for surgical resection of sinonasal papilloma. Endoscopic approaches continue to gain acceptance and become the standard of care for resection of sinonasal papillomas.

References

1. Mansell NJ, Bates GJ. The inverted Schneiderian papilloma: a review and literature report of 43 new cases. Rhinology. Sep 2000;38(3):97-101.
2. Lawson W, Nicolas F, Schlecht, Brandwein GM. The Role of the Human Papillomavirus in the Pathogenesis of Schneiderian Inverted Papillomas: An Analytic Overview of the Evidence. Head and Neck Pathol 2200; 8: 49–59.
3. Schlosser RJ, Mason JC, Gross CW. Aggressive endoscopic resection of inverted papilloma: an update. *Otolaryngol Head Neck Surg.* Jul 2001;125(1):49-53.
4. Kraft M, Simmen D, Kaufmann T, Holzmann D. Long-term results of endonasal sinus surgery in sinonasalpapillomas. Laryngoscope. Sep 2003;113(9):1541-7.
5. Nicolai P, Villaret AB, Bottazzoli M, Rossi E, Valsecchi MG. Ethmoid Adenocarcinoma--From Craniofacial to Endoscopic Resections: A Single-Institution Experience over 25 Years. Otolaryngol Head Neck Surg. Aug 2011;145(2):330-7.
6. Nicolai P, Battaglia P, Bignami M, et al. Endoscopic surgery for malignant tumors of the sinonasal tract and adjacent skull base: a 10-year experience. Am J Rhinol. May-Jun 2008;22(3):308-16. [Medline].
7. Lund V, Howard DJ, Wei WI. Endoscopic resection of malignant tumors of the nose and sinuses. Am J Rhinol. Jan-Feb 2007;21(1):89-94

EXPRESSION MECHANISM OF GLUCOCORTICOID RECEPTOR

Nobuo Ohta[1], Akihoro Ishida[1], Yusuke Suzuki[1], Kazuya Kurakami[1], Masaru Aoyagi[1], Seiji Kakehata[1]

[1]*Department of Otolaryngology, Head and Neck Surgery, Yamagata University Faculty of Medicine 2-2-2,*
Iida-nishi, Yamagata 990-9585, Japan

Keywords: glucocorticoid, glucocorticoid receptor-α, glucocorticoid receptor-β, steroid resistance

Introduction

Glucocorticoids (GCs) act by binding to a cytosolic GC receptor (GR), which is subsequently activated and is able to translocate to the nucleus. Once in the nucleus, the GR either binds to DNA and switches on the expression of anti-inflammatory genes or acts indirectly to repress the activity of a number of distinct signaling pathways such as nuclear factor (NF)-κB and activator protein (AP)-1. This latter step requires the recruitment of corepressor molecules. Importantly, this latter interaction is mutually repressive in that high levels of NF-κB and AP-1 attenuate GR function. A failure to respond may therefore result from reduced GC binding to GR, reduced GR expression, enhanced activation of inflammatory pathways, or lack of corepressor activity. These events can be modulated by oxidative stress, T-helper type 2 cytokines, or high levels of inflammatory mediators, all of which may lead to a reduced clinical outcome. Most patients with allergic rhinitis are successfully treated with conventional therapy. However, there is a small proportion of patients with allergic rhinitis, who show very poor response to high-dose and repeated GCs. GC resistance,

Address for correspondence: Dr. Nobuo Ohta, Department of Otolaryngology, Head and Neck Surgery, Yamagata University Faculty of Medicine 2-2-2, Iida-nishi, Yamagata 990-9585, Japan. Tel: 81-23-628-5380; Fax: 81-23-628-5382.
E-mail: noohta@med.id.yamagata-u.ac.jp.

Recent Advances in Rhinosinusitis and Nasal Polyposis, pp. 67-75
Edited by Hideyuki Kawauchi, Desiderio Passali, Ranko Mladina, Andrey Lopatin
and Dmytro Zabolotnyi
2015 © Kugler Publications, Amsterdam, The Netherlands

therefore, presents a profound management problem in these patients. Understanding the molecular mechanisms of GR action may lead to the development of new anti-inflammatory drugs or may reverse the relative steroid insensitivity that is characteristic of patients with these diseases.

How GC suppress allergic inflammation

Glucocorticoids (GCs) act by binding to and activating specific cytosolic GC receptors (GRs), which are held in a resting state by a number of chaperone proteins. These activated GRs then have to translocate into the nucleus before they can regulate inflammatory gene expression.[1, 2] Once in the nucleus, the activated GR can induce the expression of a number of key anti-inflammatory genes following a direct association with DNA at GC response elements (GREs) in the promoter regions of these genes. Alternatively, the activated GR can selectively repress the transcription of specific inflammatory genes without binding to DNA itself but by a number of pleiotropic actions at the promoters of inflammatory genes (Figure 1). Inflammatory genes are regulated by the actions of pro-inflammatory transcription factors such as nuclear factor (NF)-κB, activator protein (AP)-1, and signal transducer and activator of transcription proteins. Activated GR binds to these transcription factors, either directly or indirectly, and recruits corepressor proteins that blunt the ability of these transcription factors to switch on inflammatory genes.[1] GCs are commonly used as anti-inflammatory

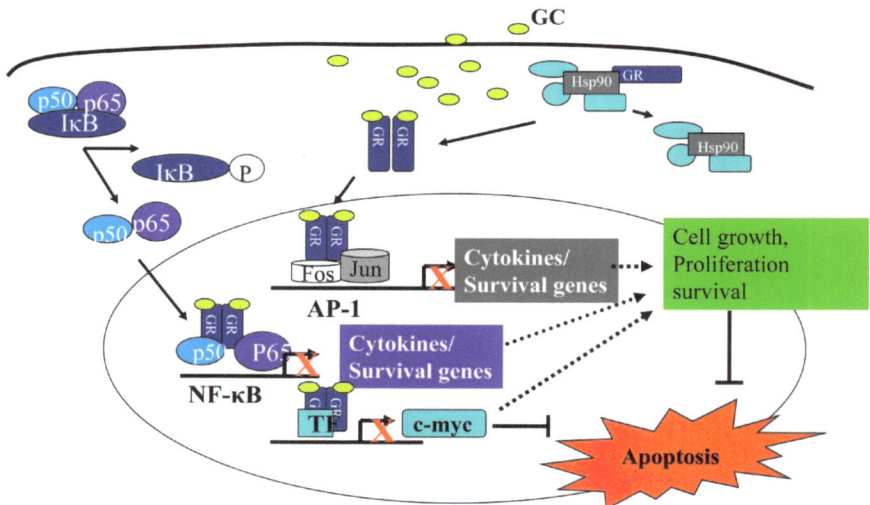

Fig. 1. Mechanism of GC action. After entering to the cytoplasm, GC bind to GR-α, associated heat-shock proteins (hsp90) are released, and the ligand-bound receptor translocates into the nucleus. A GR-α dimer bind to glucocorticoid responsive elements (GRE) on the promoter region of target genes and activate gene transcription. Protein-protein interactions between GR-α and transcription factors (NF-kB, AP-1) repress the transcription of pro-inflammatory genes.

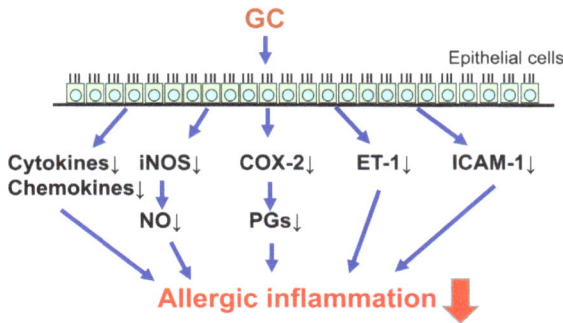

Fig. 2. Cellular mechanism of GC on epithelial cells. GC has variety of functions on respiratory epithelial cells including, cytokines, chemokines, NO production, adhesion molecules, and lead to down-regulation of the allergic inflammation.

agents in the treatment of chronic allergic diseases, including allergic rhinitis and bronchial asthma. GCs have a variety of functions, including suppressing cytokines and chemokines, down-regulating NO and prostaglandins production as well as adhesion molecules. (Figure 2) These cytokines and mediators might play important roles in regulation of allergic responses and down-regulation of these mediators lead to suppression of allergic inflammation.

Regulation of GR and isoforms

GR has two isoforms. GR-α is responsible for the induction and repression of target genes, it is expressed in virtually all human cells and tissues, and its expression is known to be down-regulated by GC[2]. GR-β is unable to bind GR. GR-β mRNA has been found to be expressed in a variety of human cells and tissues, although in much lower amount than GR-α mRNA. (Figure 3) Recent studies demonstrated that different inflammatory and immunological modulators and molecules might be involved in the regulation of GR.[3,4,5,6] (Figure 4) The results imply that down-regulation of PPARγ by cigarette smoke promotes inflammatory pathways and diminishes glucocorticoid responsiveness, thereby contributing to COPD pathogenesis, and further suggest that PPARγ agonists may be useful for COPD treatment.[6]

GC resistance in allergic rhinitis

There have been emerging advances in the understanding of molecular and cellular mechanism in GC resistance. At a molecular level, resistance to the anti-inflammatory effects of GC can be induced by several mechanisms, which may differ between patients. The reduction in the GC responsiveness observed in cells from patients with CSR asthma, asthma patients who smoke, and patients

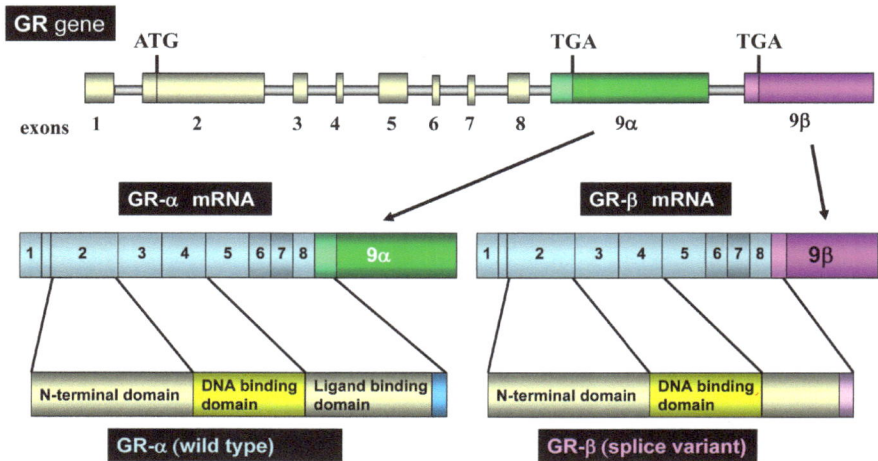

Fig. 3. Modulators of GC. Many factors might be involved in modulation of GC.

Modulators	Molecules
Ligands	11β-HSD (type1, type2), glucocorticoid agonist antagonist, SeGRM, membrane transporter
GR	GR isoform (GRβ), GR SNPs, GR mutation
Modulations	Phosphorylation, methylation, acethylation, SUMO
Chaperone	Heat shock protein, RAP46, FKBP, 14-3-3
Cofactor	Coactivator /Corepressor (CBP/p300、P160 family) SWI/SNF, DRIP/TRAP complex, FLASH
Transcription factor	NF-κB, AP-1, STATs, COUP-TF II, CREB, C/EBP Nur77, p53, GATA-1, Oct-1, NF-1
Target gene	PPARα

Fig. 4. Glucocorticoid receptor isoforms. The human GR gene is encoded on chromosome 5q31.3 and consists of nine exons. Alternative splicing of exon nine generates two receptor isoforms, GR-α and GR-β. GR-α can bind to GC, however, GR-β is lack of ligand binding domain.

with COPD has been variably ascribed to reduced GR expression, the altered affinity of the ligand for GR, the reduced ability of the GR to bind to DNA, the reduced expression and/or activity of corepressor proteins, or the increased expression of inflammatory transcription factors, such as NF-κB and AP-1.[1,2] Furthermore, unlike familial GC resistance, in which there are mutations in GR and a subsequent resetting of the basal cortisol level, these CSR patients have normal cortisol levels and do not have Addison disease. Many of these CSR asthma patients are not completely unresponsive to GCs but will respond to much higher doses than normal with the corollary that the side effects are

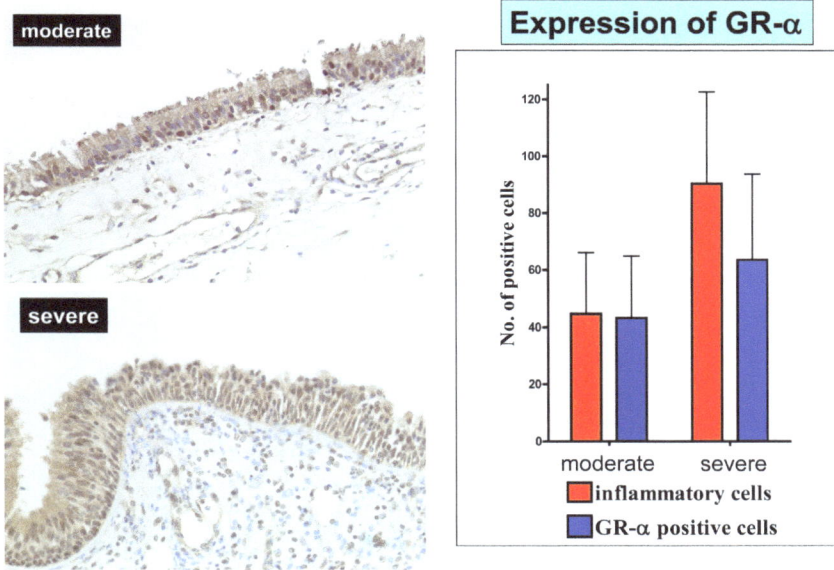

Fig. 5. Representative pathological findings of GR-α and GR-α immunoreactivities in the nasal mucosa of patients with severe nasal allergy and controls. The expression of GR-α in the nasal mucosa of patients with severe nasal allergy and controls. (original magnification ×100). (Data partially obtained from reference 24.)

increased. Alternatively, the multiple mechanisms underlying CSR asthma may indicate the need for patient-specific treatment with novel therapies directed at abnormal signaling pathways to restore asthma control.[1,2] For example, treatment with anti-IgE therapy in a small cohort of these CSR patients has shown clinical effectiveness, although the cost-effectiveness of this treatment is under debate.[7,8]

One of the factors associated with GC sensitivity is the presence of non-binding GR variants, such as GR-β. It is generally considered that interference by non-binding GR variants may result in GC resistance.[9,10,11,12,13,14] For example, GR-β expression in peripheral blood mononuclear cells increased in patients with bronchial asthma or ulcerative colitis who did not respond to GC administration.[15,16,17,18,19,20] A co-transfection assay demonstrated that GR-β inhibited GRα-mediated transcriptional signals.[20,21] These results strongly suggest that GR-β expression in inflammatory cells could influence a patient's sensitivity to GC, and explain why some patients exhibit persistent GC resistance despite high-dose treatment. The precise physiological role of GR-β remains controversial.[22,23,24] We observed significantly increased expression of GR-β in the nasal epithelium and submucosal inflammatory cells of patients with severe nasal allergy, and a significantly higher ratio of GR-β/GR-α. (Figure 5, 6, 7 and 8) Although the precise physiological role of GR-β remains elusive, GC resistance seems to be caused by insufficient GR-α, excessive GR-β, or both. GR-β might act as a negative regulator of transcription and an inhibitor of signal transduc-

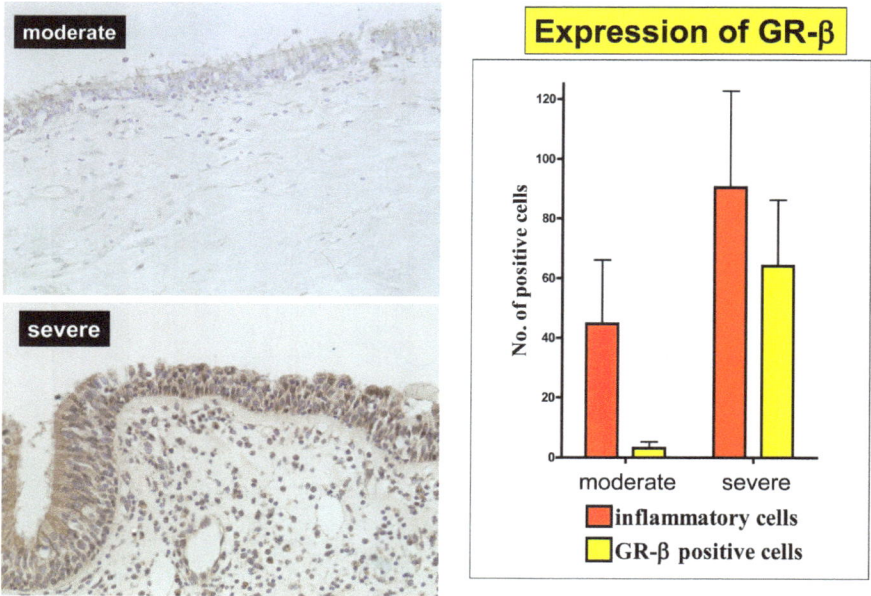

Fig. 6. Representative pathological findings of GR-β and GR-β immunoreactivities in the nasal mucosa of patients with severe nasal allergy and control. The expression of GR-β in the nasal mucosa of patients with severe nasal allergy and controls. (original magnification ×100). (Data partially obtained from reference 24.)

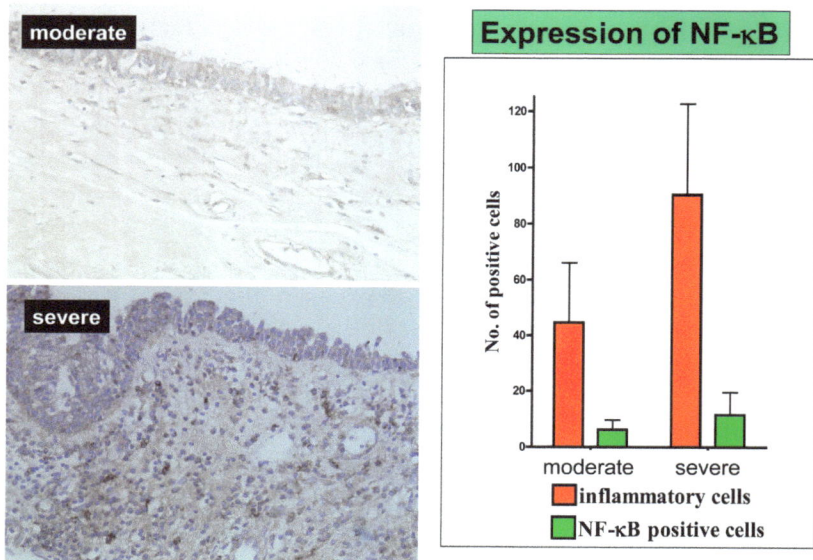

Fig. 7. Representative pathological findings of NF-kB and NF-kB immunoreactivities in the nasal mucosa of patients with severe nasal allergy and controls. The expression of NF-kB in the nasal mucosa of patients with severe nasal allergy and controls. (original magnification ×100). (Data partially obtained from reference 24.)

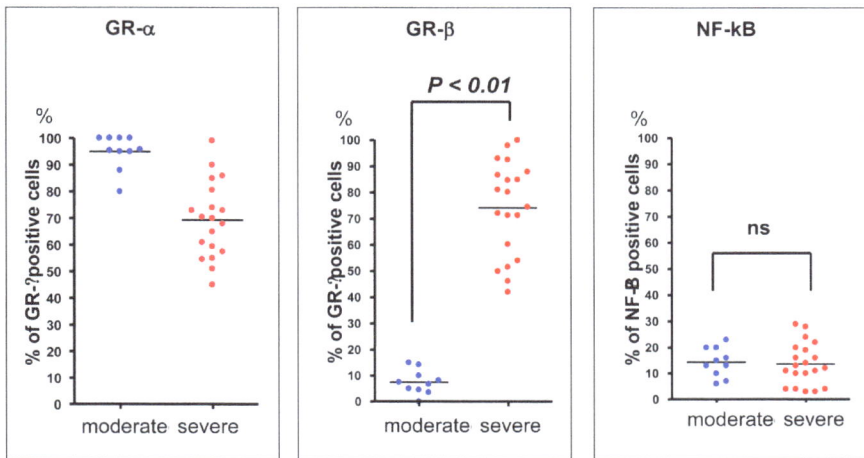

Fig. 8. The number of GR-a-, GR-b- and NF-kB-positive cells in the nasal mucosa of patients with severe nasal allergy and controls. (Data partially obtained from reference 24.)

tion. Other mechanisms have also been proposed to account for cellular steroid resistance, including overexpression of transcription factors such as NF-kB and AP-1, which antagonize GR function at the level of gene transcription and via protein–protein interactions.[22,23] NF-kB and AP-1 are induced by multiple cytokines, including TNF-a and IL-6. GR-α can also interact with other proteins regulating inflammation, such as NF-kB.[22,23] Overexpression of NF-kB caused by prolonged inflammation has been associated with GC resistance.

Conclusions

On the basis of these findings, we speculate that the amount of appearance of GR-β in the cases who need operation was significantly high compared with healthy control, and the expression of GR-β might be used as an additional parameter indicating GC resistance.

Acknowledgment

This work was supported by a Grant-in-Aid for Scientific Research (C), grant number 14571605, from the Japan Society for the Promotion of Science and the Ministry of Health, Labour and Welfare of Japan. We express our sincere thanks to Mrs. Yuko Ohta, Uyo Gakuen College, for her editorial assistance.

References

1. Trevor JL, Deshane JS. Refractory asthma: mechanisms, targets, and therapy. Allergy 2014;69(7):817-27.
2. Reddy D, Little FF Glucocorticoid-resistant asthma: more than meets the eye. J Asthma. 2013;50(10):1036-44.
3. Särndahl E, Bergström I, Nijm J, Forslund T, Perretti M, Jonasson L Enhanced neutrophil expression of annexin-1 in coronary artery disease. Metabolism. 2010 ;59(3):433-40.
4. Dezitter X, Fagart J, Taront S, Fay M, Masselot B, Hétuin D, Formstecher P, Rafestin-Oblin ME, Idziorek T Structural explanation of the effects of dissociated glucocorticoids on glucocorticoid receptor transactivation. Mol Pharmacol. 2014;85(2):226-36.
5. Murani E, Reyer H, Ponsuksili S, Fritschka S, Wimmers K M A substitution in the ligand binding domain of the porcine glucocorticoid receptor affects activity of the adrenal gland. PLoS One. 2012;7(9):e45518.
6. Lakshmi SP, Reddy AT, Zhang Y, Sciurba FC, Mallampalli RK, Duncan SR, Reddy RC Down-regulated peroxisome proliferator-activated receptor γ (PPARγ) in lung epithelial cells promotes a PPARγ agonist-reversible proinflammatory phenotype in Chronic Obstructive Pulmonary Disease (COPD). J Biol Chem. 2014 ;289(10):6383-93.
7. Thompson PJ1, Misso NL, Woods Omalizumab (Xolair) in patients with steroid-resistant asthma: lessons to be learnt. J Respirology. 2007 ; Suppl 3:S29-34.
8. Wu, AC, Paltiel, AD, Kuntz, KM, et al Cost-effectiveness of omalizumab in adults with severe asthma: results from the Asthma Policy Model. J Allergy Clin Immunol 2007;120,1146-1152.
9. Matthews JG, Ito K, Barnes PJ, Adock IM. Defective glucocorticoid receptor nuclear translocation and altered histone acetylation patterns in glucocorticoid-resistant patients. J Allergy Clin Immunol 2004;113:1100-8.
10. Okazaki S, Yamakawa M, Maeda K, Ohta N, Aoyagi M. Expression of glucocorticoid receptors in non-neoplastic lymphoid follicles and B cell type malignant lymphomas. J Clin Pathol 2006;59(4):410-6.
11. Watanabe K, Shirasaki H, Kanaizumi E, Himi T. Effects of glucocorticoids on infiltrationg cells and epithelial cells of nasal polyps. Ann Otol Rhinol Laryngol 2004;113:465-73.
12. Hamilos DL, Leung DY, Muro S, Kahn AM, Hamilos SS, Thawley SE, et al. GRb expression in nasal polyp inflammatory cells and its relationship to the anti-inflammatory effects of intranasal fluticasone. J Allergy Clin Immunol 2001;108:59-68.
13. Beppu T, Ohta N, Gon S, Sakata K, Inamura K, Fukase S, et al. Eosinophil and eosinophil cationic protein in allergic rhinitis. Acta Otolaryngol (Suppl) 1994;511:221-3.
14. Sausa AR, Lane SJ, Cidlowski JA, Staynov DZ, Lee TH. Glucocorticoid resistance in asthma is associated with elevated in vivo expression of the glucocorticoid receptor beta-isoform. J Allergy Clin Immunol 2000;105:943-50.
15. Osada R, Takeno S, Hirakawa K, Ueda T, Furukido K, Yajin K. Expression and localization of nuclear factor-kappa B subunits in cultured human paranasal sinus mucosal cells. Rhinology 2003;41(2):80-6.
16. Takeno S, Hirakawa K, Ueda T, Furukido K, Osada R, Yajin K. Nuclear factor-kappa B activation in the nasal polyp epithelium: relationship to local cytokine gene expression. Laryngoscope 2002;112(1):53-8.
17. Adcock IM, Barnes PJ. Molecular mechanisms of corticosteroid resistance. Chest 2008;134(1):394-401.
18. Meltzer EO. The pharmacological basis for the treatment of perennial allergic rhinitis and non-allergic rhinitis with topical corticosteroids. Allergy 1997;52:33-40.
19. Pullerits T, Praks L, Skoogh BE, Ani R, Lotvall J. Randomized placebo-controlled study comparing a leukotriene receptor antagonist and a nasal glucocorticoid in seasonal allergic rhinitis. Am J Respir Crit Care Med 1999;159(6):1814-8.
20. Lonqui CA, Faria CD. Evaluation of glucocorticoid sensitivity and its potential clinical applicability. Horm Res 2009;71(6):305-9.

21. Wright RJ. Stress and acquired glucocoticoid resistance:a relationship hanging in the balance. J Allergy Clin Immunol 2009;123(4):831-2.
22. Corrigan CJ, Loke TK. Clinical and molecular aspects of glucocorticoid resistant asthma. Ther Clin Risk Manag 2007;3(5):771-87.
23. Sczepankiewicz A, Breborowicz A, Sobkowiak P, Popiel A. No association of glucocorticoid receptor polymorphisms with asthma and response to glucocorticoids. Adv Med Sci 2008;52(2):245-50.
24. Ishida A, Ohta N, Koike S, Aoyagi M, Yamakawa M Overexpression of glucocorticoid receptor-beta in severe allergic rhinitis. Auris Nasus Larynx. 2010;37(5):584-8.

LAMB'S HEAD AS A MODEL FOR ENDOSCOPIC SINUS AND SKULL-BASE SURGERY (ESSBS) TRAINING

Ranko Mladina

ORL Department, Clinical Hospital Center Zagreb, Zagreb, Croatia

A lamb's head is an effective and user-friendly animal model for the first-grade education and training of the endoscopic sinus and skull base surgery (ESSBS) techniques and handling the endoscope and other instruments, before the use of expensive and disposable simulators or human cadaver models. The learning curve appeared to be quite abrupt.

We have investigated the real possibilities of training ESSBS techniques on a lamb's head, *i.e.*, on the real-tissue model, practicing the proper use and handling of the endoscope and other instruments used in everyday practice. The objective was to define the learning curve in developing ESSBS skills on the animal model.

For this purpose, five inexperienced residents performed bilateral 5-step dissections on five heads each, beginning from the inferior turbinate removal over cerebrospinal fluid leak repair to Draf III procedure. The time needed to complete particular steps as well as the whole dissection have been measured and compared to the time-standards. According to the time-standards, the duration of the whole 5-step procedure should not last longer than 24 minutes. The whole dissection performed by our inexperienced residents, however, lasted for minimally 40.5 minutes and maximally 54.5 minutes, with an average duration of 47.8 minutes.

Time rates in the residents group became shorter as they gained more experience: the fifth, final dissection took minimally 27.0 and maximally 31.0 minutes, with an average duration of 28.7 minutes!

Address for correspondence: Prof. Dr. Ranko Mladina, 10.000 Zagreb, Hrastik 11 A, Croatia. E-mail: rmladina@gmail.com

Recent Advances in Rhinosinusitis and Nasal Polyposis, p. 77
Edited by Hideyuki Kawauchi, Desiderio Passali, Ranko Mladina, Andrey Lopatin and Dmytro Zabolotnyi
2015 © Kugler Publications, Amsterdam, The Netherlands

A NOVEL SUBCLASSIFICATION FOR CHRONIC RHINOSINUSITIS WITH NASAL POLYP(S) IN JAPAN

Junichi Ishitoya, Yasunori Sakuma

Department of Otorhinolaryngology, Yokohama City University Medical Center, Yokohama, Japan

Introduction

Although chronic rhinosinusitis is a common disease, its pathophysiology remains controversial. While many etiological factors are thought to induce chronic rhinosinusitis,[1-3] a clear understanding of what triggers the pathogenesis that leads to chronic inflammation of the sinuses is still lacking. One explanation is that the pathogenesis may differ between different subtypes of chronic rhinosinusitis.

In Europe and the United States, chronic rhinosinusitis is divided into two subtypes: chronic rhinosinusitis with polyps (CRSwNP) and chronic rhinosinusitis without polyp (CRSsNP).[4,5] Most patients with CRSwNP were reported to show a strong tendency for recurrence after surgery and pronounced eosinophil infiltration in the nasal polyps.[5] In contrast, **fewer than** 50% of cases of CRSwNP in Japan and other countries in East Asia, including Korea and China, exhibit eosinophilic inflammation.[6-8] Therefore, it is necessary to distinguish these subtypes of CRSwNP in East Asia for choosing a treatment strategy.

Until 30 years ago, most CRSwNP in Japan exhibited purulent rhinorrhea, including abundant neutrophils. Thus, the inflammation of the CRSwNP was assumed to be neutrophilic. However, at the end of the 1980s, the introduction of macrolide therapy (low-dose, long-term administration of macrolide antibiotic) and the adoption of new endoscopic sinus surgery (ESS) have enabled us to successfully control the CRSwNP.[9,10] In the 1990s, macrolide therapy was established as first-line therapy, and its use in combination with ESS became the gold standard treatment for the CRSwNP in Japan.[11] After it became possible

Address for correspondence: Junichi Ishitoya, MD, PhD, Ishitoya ENT Clinic, 6-4-29-3F, Minamikarasuyama, Setagaya, Tokyo 157-0062, Japan. E-mail: ent1408@ishitoya.jp

Recent Advances in Rhinosinusitis and Nasal Polyposis, pp. 79-86
Edited by Hideyuki Kawauchi, Desiderio Passali, Ranko Mladina, Andrey Lopatin and Dmytro Zabolotnyi
2015 © Kugler Publications, Amsterdam, The Netherlands

Table 1. Comparison of clinical features between rECRS and non-rECRS

	Refractory eosinophilic chronic rhinosinusitis (rECRS)	Japanese conventional chronic rhinosinusitis (non-rECRS)
Endonasal findings	Bilateral nasal polyps, high viscous secretion	Nasal polyp in the middle meatus, mucopurulent secretion
Blood examination	Eosinophilia	–
Macrolide therapy	Not effective	Effective
Recurrent rate of nasal polyps after surgery	Very high	Low
Systemic steroid for recurrence	Higher efficacy	Unclear

to successfully control the CRSwNP, Japanese researchers began to focus on CRSwNP refractory to the combined therapy. Because one of the histological characteristics of this disease is abundant eosinophil infiltration of the nasal polyp, the term refractory eosinophilic chronic rhinosinusitis (rECRS) has been used to classify this subtype in Japan since 2001.[12]

The clinical features that differ between rECRS and Japanese conventional CRSwNP (neutrophil-dominant) are listed in Table 1.[13]

The aim of the study was to characterize the heterogeneity of CRSwNP by evaluating its clinical features and to propose a new subclassification for CRSwNP. Since allergic fungal rhinosinusitis and cystic fibrosis are uncommon in Japan, these diseases are not included in this subclassification.

Materials and methods

Patients

All subjects enrolled in this study had bilateral chronic rhinosinusitis with nasal polyp(s) (CRSwNP). A total of 111 adult patients undergoing ESS were categorized into three groups. Patients with rECRS were initially classified based on our clinical criteria for rECRS (Table 2).[13] rECRS was suspected if a patient fulfilled criteria 1, 2 and 3 in Table 2. If the patient had recurrent nasal polyps after the surgery and the polyps disappeared upon systemic steroid administration (30 mg prednisolone with a two-week dose tapering period), the diagnosis of rECRS was confirmed[14]. Thus, criterion 4 plays an important role for the final diagnosis. The remaining patients of CRSwNP were categorized with either non-refractory eosinophilic chronic rhinosinusitis with allergic rhinitis (CRSwAR) or non-refractory eosinophilic chronic rhinosinusitis without allergic rhinitis (CRSw/oAR) based on the presence or absence of perennial allergic rhinitis.

Allergic rhinitis was diagnosed according to Japanese guideline for allergic rhinitis.[15] In addition, perennial allergic rhinitis was defined as the presence of

Table 2. Clinical diagnostic indicators for rECRS

1. Characteristic clinical features
   • Bilateral nasal polyposis
2. CT scan findings (Lund-Mackay scoring system)
   • Mean ethmoid sinus scores ≥1
   • Predominant opacification of the ethmoid sinus
     (Mean ethmoid sinus scores ≥ mean maxillary sinus scores)
3. Peripheral blood eosinophil count above the normal range
4. Post-operative course
   • Strong tendency for nasal polyps recurrence after surgery
   • Effectiveness of a systemic steroid against recurrent nasal polyps

specific serum IgE(s) against perennial antigen(s) (*e.g.*, house dust mites, mold, and animal dander).

None of the patients in this study had previously undergone sinus surgery or had received any oral steroid treatments before ESS.

This study was approved by the ethics committee of the Yokohama City University Medical Center.

Clinical examinations and findings

Clinical examinations were performed as part of our routine diagnostic evaluation. Blood examinations included a complete blood count and assays for total serum IgE and specific serum IgEs against 13 common inhaled antigens. Nasal examinations were performed by endoscopy. Computed tomography (CT) scans of the sinuses were graded according to the Lund-Mackay system.[16] CT scores were expressed as the sum of the scores from both sides.

Histological eosinophilia

Nasal polyps were surgically removed, processed for histological studies, and stained with hematoxylin and eosin. Eosinophils in the lamina propria were independently counted by two of the authors in three different eosinophil-abundant fields at 400x magnification (per 0.238 mm^2). The mean count was reviewed and used as the number of infiltrated eosinophils in the nasal polyp.

Statistical analysis

The clinical findings that characterized each subtype of CRSwNP were analyzed by logistic regression analysis using SPSS software (SPSS Inc., Chicago, IL).

Results

Clinical characteristics of each subgroup

Based on our criteria, 39 patients (35.1%) were classified as rECRS, 26 (23.4%) as CRSwAR and 46 (41.4%) as CRSw/oAR. The clinical findings regarding allergic conditions for each group of patients are shown in Table 3. More than half of the patients with rECRS had asthma complications, with 12 patients (57.1%) having comorbid non-atopic asthma. rECRS patients exhibited apparent blood eosinophilia, with 13 patients (33.3%) showing high-grade blood eosinophilia that was more than twice the normal range. Blood eosinophilia was also noted in the CRSwAR group, but values were within twice the normal range in all patients.

The CT scores for each sinus in each group of patients are shown in Figure 1 and were statistically compared using logistic regression analysis. All of the clinical features examined in this study, except for the CT score of the maxillary sinus, were significantly different between rECRS and CRSw/oAR (Table 4). Although total serum IgE, comorbid asthma and CT scores of the maxillary sinus and the anterior ethmoid sinus were not significantly different between rECRS and CRSwAR, the other clinical features were significantly different

Table 3. Allergic status

	n	Asthma comorbidity	Serum total IgE (μg/ml)		Blood eosinophils (% of white blood cells)		Infiltrated eosinophils in nasal polyp (/0.238 mm²)	
			mean	*median*	*mean*	*median*	*mean*	*median*
rECRS	39	21 (53.8%)	305	196	11.1	9	444	400
CRSwAR	26	11 (42.3%)	526	282	6.2	6.5	151	66
CRSw/oAR	46	3 (6.5%)	109	50	3.8	2.7	87	12.4

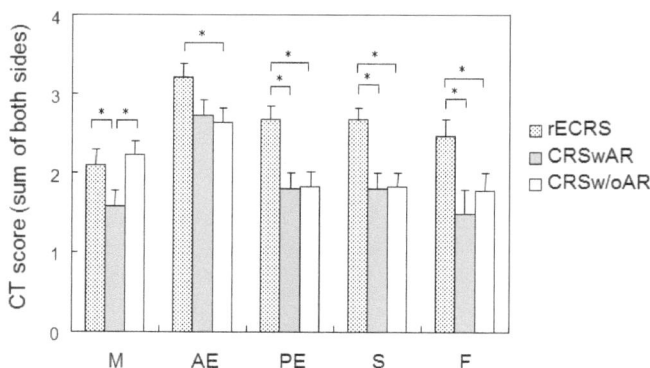

*Statistically significant; error bars: standard error; M: maxillary sinus; AE: anterior ethmoid sinus; PE: posterior ethmoid sinus; S: sphenoid sinus; F: frontal sinus.

Table 4. Odds ratios for clinical findings: rECRS vs. CRSw/oAR

	Odds ratio	95% confidence limit		*p*
		Lower	Upper	
Peripheral blood eosinophils (%)	*1.70*	*1.35*	*2.14*	*<0.001*
Total serum IgE (/100)	*1.65*	*1.22*	*2.22*	*0.002*
Asthma (1)	*16.72*	*4.42*	*63.16*	*<0.001*
Eosinophil infiltration in the nasal polyp (number/50)	*1.42*	*1.22*	*1.64*	*<0.001*
CT findings (scores)				
Maxillary	0.92	0.64	1.32	0.654
Anterior ethmoid	*2.00*	*1.20*	*3.32*	*0.008*
Posterior ethmoid	*1.88*	*1.40*	*2.86*	*0.003*
Sphenoid	*1.65*	*1.20*	*2.26*	*0.002*
Frontal	*1.41*	*1.03*	*1.94*	*0.032*

Table 5. Odds ratios for clinical findings: rECRS vs. CRSwAR

	Odds ratio	95% confidence limit		*p*
		Lower	Upper	
Peripheral blood eosinophils (%)	*1.36*	*1.13*	*1.63*	*0.001*
Total serum IgE (/100)	0.90	0.82	1.00	0.125
Asthma (1)	1.59	0.59	4.33	0.363
Eosinophil infiltration in the nasal polyp (number/50)	*1.35*	*1.16*	*1.57*	*<0.001*
CT findings (scores)				
Maxillary	1.51	0.96	2.39	0.077
Anterior ethmoid	1.74	1.00	3.30	0.05
Posterior ethmoid	*2.21*	*1.27*	*3.86*	*0.005*
Sphenoid	*1.80*	*1.21*	*2.67*	*0.004*
Frontal	*1.59*	*1.10*	*2.29*	*0.013*

(Table 5). Meanwhile, there were no significant differences in CT scores between CRSwAR and CRSw/oAR, except for the maxillary sinus (Table 6). When differences were observed between these two subgroups, they were generally related to allergic conditions associated with blood eosinophils, total serum IgE and asthma comorbidity (Tables 3, 6).

Pathophysiological features

The extent of tissue eosinophilia in the nasal polyp differed between each subtype of CRSwNP (Table 3); rECRS showed marked tissue eosinophilia, while CRSwAR and CRSw/oAR exhibited mild and minor tissue eosinophilia, respectively. The number of infiltrating eosinophils in the nasal polyp was

Table 6. Odds ratios for clinical findings: CRSwAR vs. CRSw/oAR

	Odds ratio	95% confidence limit		p
		Lower	Upper	
Peripheral blood eosinophils (%)	1.21	1.05	1.40	0.010
Total serum IgE (/100)	1.82	1.22	2.70	0.002
Asthma (1)	10.51	2.58	42.86	0.001
Eosinophil infiltration in the nasal polyp (number/50)	1.12	0.95	1.22	0.171
CT findings (scores)				
Maxillary	0.61	0.39	0.96	0.031
Anterior ethmoid	1.11	0.68	1.83	0.674
Posterior ethmoid	0.99	0.66	1.48	0.949
Sphenoid	0.91	0.63	1.33	0.633
Frontal	0.87	0.62	1.22	0.426

significantly greater in patients with rECRS than in patients with CRSwAR or CRSw/oAR (Tables 4, 5).

Discussion

CRSwNP in Japan is more heterogeneous compared with CRSwNP in Western countries. Until 1980s, most Japanese CRSwNP patients exhibited neutrophil-dominant inflammation and the combination of both macrolide therapy and ESS was very effective for these patients. However, CRSwNP with eosinophil-dominant inflammation which was very refractory to the combination treatment has gradually increased and this subtype has been called as refractory eosinophilic chronic rhinosinusitis (rECRS) in Japan since 2001.[12] Because therapeutic strategies for these subtypes of CRSwNP are different each other (Table 1), it has become increasingly important to be able to differentiate rECRS from non-rECRS before initiating therapy.

The nasal polyps in patients with perennial allergic rhinitis also exhibit eosinophilic infiltration and the differences between rECRS and CRSwAR have been sometimes confused. However, because CRSwAR does not usually exhibit a strong tendency to recur after surgery, this subtype should be distinguished from rECRS. Therefore, we diagnosed rECRS first by its characteristic clinical feature[14] and the rest of CRSwNP was categorized into CRSwAR and CRSw/oAR according to with or without perennial allergic rhinitis. Then, we compared the clinical and pathophysiological features between these three subtypes of CRSwNP.

We found that CT scores were significantly different between rECRS and CRSw/oAR and between rECRS and CRSwAR (Tables 4, 5). In contrast, except for the maxillary sinus, there were no differences in CT scores between

CRSwAR and CRSw/oAR (Table 6). Thus, the opacity of the sinus CT image in rECRS appears to be different from that in CRSwAR and CRSw/oAR. The most characteristic CT finding for rECRS appears to be the involvement of the posterior ethmoid sinus.

The ostiomeatal complex (OMC) was reported to play a fundamental role in the pathogenesis of chronic rhinosinusitis, and impaired ostial patency was thought to be a key element in chronic sinus inflammation.[13] The sinuses that are most likely to be affected by this pathogenesis are the maxillary sinus, anterior ethmoid sinus and the sinus cells that connect to the middle meatus (anterior group of paranasal sinus). In fact, the CT score for the anterior ethmoid sinus was much higher than that of the posterior ethmoid sinus in CRSwAR and CRSw/oAR, while the CT scores for the posterior ethmoid sinus and sphenoid sinus were significantly higher in rECRS than in other CRSwNP. These data suggest that the pathogenesis of rECRS differs from that of CRSwAR and CRSw/oAR and that the pathological changes in the OMC might be less important in the pathogenesis of rECRS. Although the reason why rECRS affects posterior groups of paranasal sinus more likely is unclear, edematous change of middle turbinate might be important for it.

Prominent tissue and blood eosinophilia is a distinct feature of rECRS. While CRSwAR also showed tissue and blood eosinophilia, the extent of eosinophilia is less severe than that in rECRS. Among patients with rECRS and comorbid asthma, comorbid asthma was of the non-atopic type in more than half of these cases (12 of 21 patients; data not shown) and the total serum IgE of rECRS was lower than that in CRSwAR. These data suggest that the prominent tissue and blood eosinophilia of rECRS might be independent of serum IgE and other IgE-independent molecules may play an important role in inducing eosinophilic inflammation.

However, what are the differences between CRSwAR and CRSw/oAR? The opacity of sinus CT images for CRSwAR was similar to that for CRSw/oAR, except in the maxillary sinus. In CRSwAR, nasal allergy induces a diffuse swelling of the nasal mucosa, making it easier for the ethmoid sinus to be affected because of the smaller ostia. Our gene expression study did not show any apparent differences between CRSwAR and CRSw/oAR, which suggests that there are no essential differences in pathophysiology between these subtypes, except for the presence or absence of nasal allergy (data not shown). The presence of nasal allergy in these patients might influence the clinical features, including comorbid asthma.

Macrolide therapy, which is treatment with low-dose, long-term 14-membered ring macrolides, was found to be effective for diffuse panbronchiolitis (DPB) in Japan in 1984. This treatment was also reported to be effective for chronic sinusitis which was associated with DPB and reported efficacy of macrolide therapy was 60-70% for CRSwNP patients showing neutrophil-dominant inflammation. However, the macrolide therapy is not effective for rECRS. Therefore, differential diagnosis of CRSwNP is very important before choosing the treatment for CRSwNP.

In conclusion, we have proposed a novel subclassification for CRSwNP, namely rECRS and other subtypes. The latter may have small variations in disease characteristics, and can be further classified as CRSwAR and CRSw/oAR. The use of this new subclassification should help us to better use the currently available therapeutic options and assist with planning of clinical studies in Japan and East Asia. These results might also be applicable to Caucasian patients with CRSwNP.

References

1. Rudack C, Sachse FA, lberty J. Chronic rhinosinusitis need for further classification? Inflamm Res 2004;53:111-117.
2. Ferguson BJ. Categorization of eosinophilic chronic rhinosinusitis. Curr Opin Otolaryngol Head Neck Surg 2004;12:237-242.
3. Pawliczak R, Lewandowska-Polak A, Kowalski ML. Pathogenesis of nasal polyps: an update. Curr Allergy Asthma Rep 2005;5:463-471.
4. Meltzer EO, Hamilos DL, Hadley JA, et al. Rhinosinusitis: developing guidance for clinical trials. J Allergy Clin Immunol 2006;118:S17-61.
5. Fokkens W, Lund V, Mullol J, et al. European position paper on rhinosinusitis and nasal polyps 2012. Rhinol 2012;50:Suppl 23.
6. Kim JW, Hong SL, Kim YK, et al. Histological and immunological features of non-eosinophilic nasal polyps. Otolaryngol Head Neck Surg 2007;137:925-930.
7. Zhang N, Van Zele T, Perez-Novo C, et al. Different types of T-effector cells orchestrate mucosal inflammation in chronic sinus disease. J Allergy Clin Immunol 2008;122:961-968.
8. Cao PP, Li HB, Wang BF, et al. Distinct immunopathologic characteristics of various types of chronic rhinosinusitis in adult Chinese. J Allergy Clin Immunol 2009;124:478-484.
9. Ichimura K, Shimazaki Y, Ishibashi T, et al. Effect of new macrolide roxithromycin upon nasal polyps associated with chronic sinusitis. Auris Nasus Larynx 1996;23:48-56.
10. Kimura N, Nishioka K, Nishizaki K, et al. Clinical effect of low-dose, long-term roxithromycin chemotherapy in patients with chronic sinusitis. Acta Med Okayama 1997;51:33-37.
11. Moriyama H, Yanagi K, Ohtori N, et al. Evaluation of endoscopic sinus surgery for chronic sinusitis: post-operative erythromycin therapy. Rhinology 1995;33:166-170.
12. Haruna S, Ohtori N, Yanagi K. Eosinophilic sinusitis. Oto-Rhino-Laryngology Tokyo (in Japanese) 2001;44:195-201.
13. Ishitoya J, Sakuma Y, Tsukuda M. Eosinophilic Chronic rhinosinusitis in Japan. Allergology International 2010;59:239-245.
14. Sakuma Y, Ishitoya J, Komatsu M, et al. New clinical diagnostic criteria for eosinophilic chronic shinosinusitis. Auris Nasus Larynx 2011;38:239-245.
15. Okubo K, Kurono Y, Fujieda S, et al. Japanese Guideline for Allergic Rhinitis 2014. Allergology International 2014;63:357-375.
16. Lund V, Kennedy D. Staging for rhinosinusitis. Otolaryngol Head Neck Surg 1997;117:S35-40.

CORTICOSTEROID SENSITIVITY IN NATURAL HELPER CELLS

Koichiro Asano[1], Hiroki Kabata[2], Kazuyo Moro[3], Shigeo Koyasu[3]

[1]*Division of Pulmonary Medicine, Tokai University School of Medicine, Kanagawa, Japan;* [2]*Division of Pulmonary Medicine, Keio University School of Medicine, Tokyo, Japan;* [3]*RIKEN Center for Integrative Medical Sciences, Yokohama, Japan*

Allergic host defence

Immunoglobulin E (IgE) and T_H2 cells are the cardinal system to eliminate macroparasites, mediating the degranulation of mast cells to release histamines and other mediators and the recruitment and activation of inflammatory cells such as eosinophils. Allergy has therefore been considered as an immune reaction against wrong targets 'allergens' such as dust mites, pollen, animal dander, fungi and others. However, allergic diseases also occur not only in the organs susceptible to parasite infection such as the intestines and colons, but also in the eyes, upper and lower airways, and skins where parasite infection is rare. The common feature of these organs is the presence of epithelial interface that separates the environment and the body. Medzhitov and colleagues[1] proposed a new concept on allergy, 'allergic host defences', stating that "allergic immunity has an important role in host defence against noxious environmental substances, … appropriately targeted allergic reactions are beneficial, although they can become detrimental when excessive."[1] This concept fits well to the observation that allergic diseases occur at the organs that directly contact with the environment. If allergic reaction is truly a host defense mechanism, there should be an immune system for innate type-2 response or 'innate allergy' in addition to the system for acquired immunity such as IgE and T_H2 cells.

Address for correspondence: Koichiro Asano, MD, Division of Pulmonary Medicine, Department of Medicine, Tokai University School of Medicine, 143 Shimokasuya, Isehara, Kanagawa 259-1193, Japan. E-mail: ko-asano@tokai-u.jp

Recent Advances in Rhinosinusitis and Nasal Polyposis, pp. 87-91
Edited by Hideyuki Kawauchi, Desiderio Passali, Ranko Mladina, Andrey Lopatin and Dmytro Zabolotnyi
2015 © Kugler Publications, Amsterdam, The Netherlands

Cytokines and cells mediating innate allergy

The first clue for the presence of innate allergic response was provided in 2001, showing that IL-25 administered in mice induces the expression of type-2 cytokines (IL-4, IL-5, IL-13) and increases the number of peripheral blood eosinophils.[2] IL-33, intranasally administered, also causes eosinophil accumulation, goblet cell hyperplasia of the epithelium, and hyperresponsiveness in the airway. Type-2 immune responses induced by IL-25/IL-33 are preserved in T and B cell-deficient mice, and independent of basophils, mast cells, NK cells, but are diminished in *Rag2⁻/⁻Il2rg⁻/⁻* mice, suggesting an unidentified innate immune cell population.

In 2010, Moro *et al.*[3] reported new lymphoid cells present in lymphoid clusters of the mesenteric fat tissue (FALC). The newly-identified lymphoid cells, named as natural helper (NH) cells, produce large quantities of IL-5 and IL-13 in response to IL-25/IL-33, but lack any known lineage markers for hematopoietic cells and lymphocytes. NH cells constitutively express IL-25 and IL-33 receptors as well as IL-2 and IL-7 receptors, and present in *Rag2⁻/⁻* mice, but absent in *Rag2⁻/⁻Il2rg⁻/⁻* mice. Following this report, similar lymphoid cells such as nuocytes and innate helper type 2 cells have been reported, and these cells including NH cells are now classified as group 2 innate lymphoid cells (ILC2s).

Corticosteroid sensitivity in natural helper cells

Inhaled corticosteroids are the key drug in the treatment of asthma, as they suppress airway inflammation most robustly, however, ~5% of patients with severe/refractory asthma respond poorly to high-dose inhaled corticosteroid. We examined corticosteroid sensitivity of NH cells *in vivo* and *in vitro* to elucidate the role of innate type-2 immunity in the pathophysiology of severe asthma.[4] Effects of dexamethasone on IL-33-dependent airway inflammation were evaluated to examine *in-vivo* sensitivity of NH cells. Dexamethasone at a dose of five mg/kg body weight completely suppressed the IL-33-induced accumulation of eosinophils and lung NH cells, IL-5 and IL-13 production in the lungs, and goblet-cell hyperplasia. *In-vitro* sensitivity was examined with NH cells isolated from FALC; dexamethasone (10^{-9} M-10^{-6} M) efficiently suppressed proliferation and induced apoptosis of NH cells in a dose-dependent manner. These results confirm that NH cells are sensitive to corticosteroids *in vitro* and *in vivo*.

Mechanisms for natural helper cells to acquire corticosteroid resistance

Interestingly, IL-33-dependent airway inflammation became resistant to corticosteroids in asthmatic animals sensitized and exposed to allergen such as ovalbumin (Fig. 1). Flowcytometric analysis demonstrated that the treatment

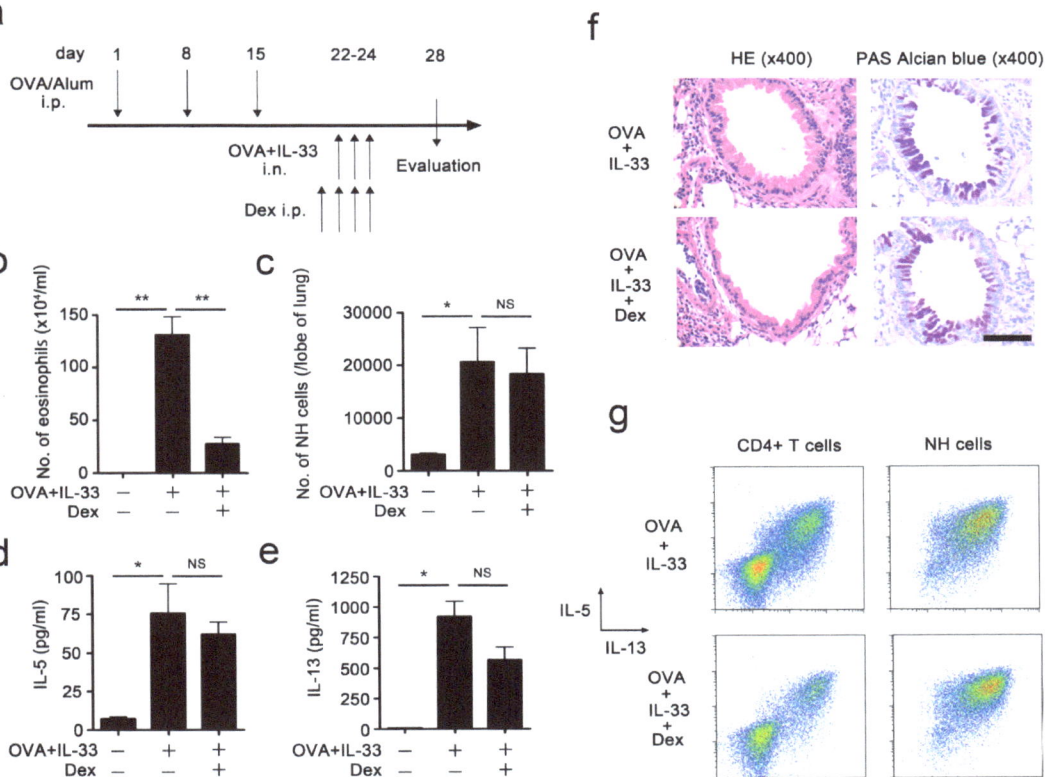

Fig. 1. Administration of IL-33 in asthma model mice (a) induces corticosteroid-resistant airway inflammation. The mice sensitized with ovalbumin (OVA) and alum were treated by intranasal administration of OVA (10 μg) and IL-33 (0.1 μg) for three consecutive days. Dexamethasone (DEX, 5 mg/kg) was intraperitoneally injected prior to OVA/IL-33 administration for some mice. Number of eosinophils in the bronchoalveolar lavage fluid (BALF, b) and NH cells in the lungs (c), amounts of IL-5 (d) and IL-13 (e) in BALF were examined four days after the final administration of OVA/IL-33. Mean ± SEM, n = 3-4 for each group. NS: not significant. *P < 0.05, **P < 0.01. (f) Representative histology of the airways from these mice stained with he-matoxylin and eosin (left panels) or periodic acid–Schiff (PAS)-alcian blue (right panels). Scale bar indicates 100 μm. (g) Intracellular staining of IL-5 and IL-13 in CD4+ T cells and NH cells. (Reproduced from ref. 4 with permission.)

with dexamethasone decreased the number of IL-5- or IL-13-positive T cells, but failed to suppress the number of NH cells or the production of T_H2 cytokines (Fig. 1f). We therefore hypothesized that there is a factor(s) in the inflammatory milieu of the allergen-exposed airways that can induce corticosteroid resistance in NH cells. We examined a panel of 15 cytokines including interleukins, TSLP, and TNF-α on isolated NH cells (Fig. 2), and found that IL-2, IL-7, IL-9, or TSLP significantly inhibited the decrease in the number of NH cells in the presence of dexamethasone (10^{-8} M). We confirmed that TSLP is responsible

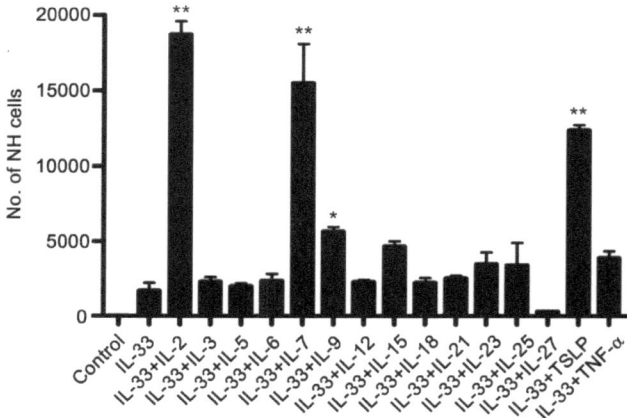

Fig. 2. Screening of cytokines that modify the corticosteroid sensitivity of NH cells. NH cells (5,000 cells/well) derived from fat-associated lymphoid cluster were cultured with IL-33 (10 ng/ml) ± various cytokines (10 ng/ml) for four days in the presence of dexamethasone (10^{-8} M). Numbers of viable (propidium iodide-negative) cells were determined using flow cytometry. Mean ± SEM, n = 3 for each group. *P < 0.05, **P < 0.01 compared to IL-33 alone. (Reproduced from ref. 4 with permission.)

for the induction of corticosteroid resistance in the asthmatic airways, based on the facts that: 1) TSLP is synthesized and released in the asthmatic airways; 2) IL-33-dependent airway inflammation acquires corticosteroid resistance in the presence of TSLP; 3) The blockade of TSLP either with a neutralizing antibody against TSLP or genetic deletion of TSLP receptor can restore the corticosteroid sensitivity in allergen/IL-33-dependent airway inflammation.

We then confirmed that STAT5 is activated in TSLP-stimulated NH cells and inhibition of STAT5 with a specific inhibitor concentration-dependently restores the effects of corticosteroid to induce apoptosis of NH cells even in the presence of TSLP. Nelson and colleagues[5] performed a high throughput screening of 1,120 clinically used drugs, and identified pimozide, a drug for the treatment of schizophrenia and other chronic neuropsychiatric diseases, as a potent STAT5 inhibitor. We proved that pimozide effectively reverses TSLP-induced corticosteroid resistance in NH cells either *in vitro* and *in vivo*.

A new perspective in the treatment of severe asthma

We have demonstrated that, although by itself sensitive to corticosteroids, the IL-33/NH cell pathway becomes resistant to corticosteroids *in vitro* and *in vivo* in the presence of TSLP, which is likely to be produced in bronchial epithelial cells of the inflamed asthmatic airways. It has recently been demonstrated that an anti-TSLP antibody effectively suppresses early- and late-asthmatic response to inhaled allergen in the patients with established asthma[6], and the antibody is currently under phase 2 clinical trial. Our data suggest the possibility that anti-TSLP drugs such as anti-TSLP antibodies and inhibitors of is signals such as pimozide can provide a new therapeutic approach in corticosteroid-resistant, severe asthma.

References

1. Palm NW, Rosenstein RK, Medzhitov R. Allergic host defences. Nature 2012;484:465-472.
2. Fort MM, Cheung J, Yen D, et al. IL-25 induces IL-4, IL-5, and IL-13 and Th2-associated pathologies in vivo. Immunity 2001;15:985-995.
3. Moro K, Yamada T, Tanabe M, et al. Innate production of T_H2 cytokines by adipose tissue-associated c-Kit$^+$Sca-1$^+$ lymphoid cells. Nature 2010;463:540-544.
4. Kabata H, Moro K, Fukunaga K, et al. Thymic stromal lymphopoietin induces corticosteroid resistance in natural helper cells during airway inflammation. Nat Commun 2013;4:2675.
5. Nelson EA, Walker SR, Weisberg E, et al. The STAT5 inhibitor pimozide decreases survival of chronic myelogenous leukemia cells resistant to kinase inhibitors. Blood 2011;117:3421-3429.
6. Gauvreau GM, O'Byrne PM, Boulet LP, et al. Effects of an anti-TSLP antibody on allergen-induced asthmatic responses. N Engl J Med 2014;370:2102-2110.

ENDOSCOPIC SINUS SURGERY FOR CHRONIC RHINOSINUSITIS – CURRENT CONCEPT AND TECHNIQUE FOR SAFE AND EFFECTIVE OPERATION

Nobuyoshi Otori

Department of Otorhinolaryngology, Jikei University School of Medicine, Tokyo, Japan

Introduction

Endoscopic sinus surgery (ESS) has become widespread as a standard surgical method for chronic rhinosinisitis (CRS). With the development of various surgical devices such as microdebrider and navigation system, ESS became safer and more adequate compared with conventional sinus operations such as the Caldwell-Luc procedure. Application of ESS is now widely extended to mucoceles, sinonasal tumors, intra-orbital diseases and skull base diseases.

The outcome of ESS for CRS has been further improved by employing postoperative low-dose long-term macrolide therapy. On the other hand, certain cases of CRS characterized by significant eosinophile infiltration to sinus mucosa and/or mucosal polyp and diagnosed as eosinophilic chronic rhinosinusitis (ECRS) are now increasing.[1] In this type of CRS, recurrence of mucosal lesion accompanied by recurrent nasal polyposis is often observed, so it is considered as persistent CRS. It is difficult to cure ECRS by ESS alone. A combination of medical and local treatment, *e.g.*, local and systemic steroids, anti-allergic agents as well as frequent sinus rinsing, is required.

Address for correspondence: Department of Otorhinolaryngology, Jikei University School of Medicine. 3-25-8, Nishishinbashi, Minato-ku, Tokyo, 105-8461, Japan. Tel: +81 3 3433 1111. Email: otori@jikei.ac.jp

Recent Advances in Rhinosinusitis and Nasal Polyposis, pp. 93-97
Edited by Hideyuki Kawauchi, Desiderio Passali, Ranko Mladina, Andrey Lopatin and Dmytro Zabolotnyi
2015 © Kugler Publications, Amsterdam, The Netherlands

Complications

Radical and thorough as well as appropriate removal of the sinus pathology leads to the patient's recovery from the diseases. On the other hand, inappropriate and rough manipulation during the surgery may cause major complications such as orbital injury and cerebrospinal fluid (CSF) leakage. Especially, prevalence of orbital injury resulting in permanent orbital dysfunction has been increasing.[2]

Key points for safer and proper surgery are:

1. Understand the anatomy, especially the anatomical relations of basal lamellas and ethmoidal air cells;
2. Examine the pre-op CT, then image a '3D'-structure;
3. Keep a clear and proper field of endoscopic view;
4. Make a suitable choice of instruments.

Forceps for safer and proper manipulation

The selection of forceps is important, not only for a safe and accurate operation, but also for obtaining good results postoperatively. There are many types of forceps, but through-cutting forceps are primarily used. They are preferred for effective preservation of mucosa and for prevention of injury. Morphologically, the orbit and brain are separated from the paranasal sinuses by a paper-thin bone wall, and sometimes part of these bony separations will show dehiscence. Therefore, pulling the mucosa, lamella, and the bone plate with cup-type forceps can be very dangerous.

Mucosal preservation

Excision of mucosa is to be avoided as much as possible. For reversible pathologic changes, diseased mucosa is preserved and its normalization through improvement in aeration and drainage is awaited.[3] For irreversible lesions showing severe edema and hypertrophy, subepithelial lesions are excised with a cutting instrument, and the mucoperiosteum is left intact (exposure of the bone surface is to be avoided). With this method, the inflammation of preserved subepithelial tissue disappears, and healthy mucosal epithelium is regenerated. The original paranasal cavity is to be maintained.

When the bone surface is exposed as a result of elimination of the mucosa and periosteum, edematous tissue first covers the exposed bone surface and soon undergoes scarring. In such tissue, regeneration of mucosal epithelium is delayed, and a long period of time is required for tissue to be covered with mucosal epithelium that extends from that surrounding. Mucosal epithelium that regenerates after elimination of all mucosa has only a small number of ciliated cells, and therefore its excretory function is poor. A thin connective tissue should be left on the bone surface; the peripheral bony boundary surface should not be exposed by any means. Such treatment facilitates ciliated epithelialization of mucosa, and recovery of the ciliary function should occur.

Surgical techniques

Ethmoidal surgery

Understanding of the location of uncinate process, bulla ethmoidalis, ground lamellae and superior turbinate is important since they serve as an anatomic landmark during the operation. The bone septa in the ethmoid air cells are sufficiently excised to make them as smooth as possible, and a unique cavity is created. Remaining ethmoid air cells are considered to be the focus of persistent and/or recurrent sinusitis.[4]

Maxillary surgery

The maxillary sinus is inspected with a 70-degree endoscopy, then a curved forceps is inserted through the fontanelle and a control hole made through the inferior nasal meatus when necessary.

Sphenoidal surgery

If possible, the sphenoid sinus should be entered from the posterior ethmoid sinus. However, when pneumatization of the sphenoid sinus is poor or an orientation of the surgical field is indistinct, it is preferable to enter from the natural ostium. Pathological lesions in the sphenoid sinus should be removed, but it is not preferable to forcibly remove a mucosal lesion from the lateral or posterior wall.

Frontal surgery

The approach to the frontal sinus lesion is the most difficult step in ESS because of the risk of complications.

1. Examine the pre-op CT-scan to image the anatomy around the drainage pathway of the frontal sinus. Especially, anatomical relations of air cells in the frontal-ethmoidal area, such as agger nasi cells, frontal ethmoidal cells, frontal bulla cells and suprabullar cells, should be examined;
2. Use a 70-degree endoscope to look up at frontal recess from below;
3. Identify the location of the lamina papyracea and the skull base which are 'danger zones', and simultaneously identify the location of the frontal recess

which should be operated. Then, inside the frontal recess, recognize the drainage pathway;

4. Manipulate the anterior part of the frontal recess by the use of angled forceps so as to prevent skull-base injury;
5. After having identified the drainage pathway, insert the angled forceps carefully into the frontal sinus, enlarging the pathway as much as possible;
6. Draf type III and Draf type II are chosen for revision surgery or in cases of short anterior-posterior diameter.

Revision ESS

Causes of recurrence of CRS may be:

1. Residual air cells and adhesions in the ethmoid area;
2. Insufficient enlargement of the ventilation and drainage pathway between the nasal cavity and sinuses;
3. Failure of mucosal preservation surgery;
4. Insufficient post-op care;
5. Post-op stenosis and/or closure of the ostia;
6. Post-op infection of the sinus mucosa;
7. Eosinophile infiltration in the sinus mucosa.

The key point of revision surgery is to create a wide communication between the sinuses. Remove the mucosal lesion by the use of through-cutting forceps or microdebrider, but avoid removing the whole mucosa from a bony surface. Periodical and long-term post-op follow-up is required.

In the case of revision surgery for CRS, disappearance and/or deformation of anatomical landmarks is often seen. Therefore, revision surgery is technically more difficult than initial surgery. Especially, how much of the turbinate and agger nasi remains determines the degree of difficulty. Friendly landmarks for proper orientation during revision surgery are:

1. The arch formed by the posterior edge of the lacrimal bone;
2. The anterior-superior attachment of the middle turbinate;
3. The middle meatal antrostomy and the ridge along its superior border formed by the floor of the orbit;
4. The lamina papyracea;
5. The nasal septum;
6. The arch of the posterior choana.

Additionally, the surgeon should carefully check the preoperative CT-scan to understand morphological changes as well as lesion in the sinuses.

Post-operative care

Although ESS removes morbid mucosal epithelium, the lamina propria and muco-periostium are saved. It is, therefore, marked as mucosal preservation surgery. On the other hand, ESS may not remove a pathological change thoroughly. Recurrence of pathological changes, such as a polyposis and mucosal edema, sometimes takes place. In the early stage after ESS, granulation is easily formed by bacterial colonization and/or infection on account of exposure of subepithelial tissue. Granulation may cause postoperative adhesion in a later stage. Moreover, the mucosal drainage function is weak until cilia are reproduced at an epithelium. Then, secretion and mucus may store in the sinuses, resulting in local recurrence of the mucosal infection. Therefore, appropriate postoperative care is necessary to attain a smooth mucosal healing process.

The key points of early-stage postoperative medical care are:

1. Prevent dryness of the surgical wound.
2. Rinse out secretion, blood and crusts from the sinuses.
3. Prevent bacterial infection of the wound.

When an evident mucosal swelling or edema is persistent, topical steroids together with low doses of an oral steroid and low-dose macrolide treatment are employed. Especially in a patient who has an allergic background such as bronchial asthma, the use of steroids is effective. When the purulent secretion accumulates in the sinus, antibiotics will be prescribed.

Recently, we began to use calcium alginate as an absorbent packing material that shows a potent hemostatic effect and is able to maintain wound surfaces in a moist environment by absorbing and gelling the wound exudate.[5] Good wound healing can be expected due to the maintenance of a moist environment.

References

1. Nakayama T, Yoshikawa M, Asaka D, et al. Mucosal eosinophilia and recurrence of nasal polyps – new classification of chronic rhinosinusitis. Rhinology 2011;49:392-396.
2. Asaka D, Nakayama T, Hama T, et al. Risk factors for complications of endoscopic sinus surgery for chronic rhinosinusitis. Am J Rhinol Allergy 2012;26:61-64.
3. Moriyama H, Yanagi K, Ohtori N, Asai K, Fukami M. Healing process of sinus mucosa after endoscopic sinus surgery. Am J Rhinol 1996;10:61-66.
4. Okushi T, Mori E, Nakayama T, et al. Impact of residual ethmoidal cells on postoperative course after endoscopic sinus surgery for chronic rhinosinusitis. Auris Nasus Larynx 2012;39:484-489.
5. Okushi T, Yoshikawa M, Otori N, et al. Evaluation of symptoms and QOL with calcium alginate versus chitin-coated gauze for middle meatus packing after endoscopic sinus surgery. Auris Nasus Larynx 2011;39:31-37.

FUNCTIONAL CHARACTERIZATION OF A SMOKE-INDUCED LONG NON-CODING RNA, SCAL1, IN PROTECTING AIRWAY EPITHELIAL CELL INJURY

Sarah N. Statt, Philip Thai, Reen Wu

Center for Comparative Respiratory Biology and Medicine, University of California at Davis, Davis, CA 95616, USA

Thanks to the boom of new sequencing technologies in the last ten years, many new non-coding RNA species are being discovered.[1] Through work completed in the last ten years, these ncRNAs are being shown to be key players in many biological processes, such as development, cell cycle regulation and post-transcriptional processing of mRNA.[2] Currently, non-coding RNAs have mainly been classified arbitrarily based on size; ncRNAs smaller than 200 bps are referred to as small ncRNAs and anything larger than 200 bps are referred to as long ncRNAs.[3] Long ncRNAs or lncRNAs have been loosely further classified based on their relative distance to coding genes: native antisense transcripts (NATs) overlap with coding genes, intronic lncRNAs are found inside introns of genes and long intergenic non-coding RNAs (lincRNAs) are found in the genomic deserts between genes.[4] Like mRNAs, lncRNAs are transcribed by RNA polymerase II and contain a polyadenylated tail. They are commonly spliced into a mature transcript form and are associated with histone signatures similar to known actively transcribed protein-coding genes: trimethylation of histone 3 lysine 4 (H3K4me3) at the transcriptional start site (TSS) and trimethylation of histone 3 lysine 36 (H3K36me3) throughout the gene body.[5] Many further classifications of lncRNAs have been proposed but have not been as widely adopted: transcribed ultraconserved regions (T-UCRs), enhancer RNAs (eRNAs), repeat-associated ncRNAs, long intronic ncRNAs, antisense RNAs, promoter-associated long RNAs and long stress-induced non-coding transcripts.[6] LncRNAs, unlike the well-characterized field of microRNAs, are a more recent

Address for correspondence: E-mail: rwu@ucdavis.edu

Recent Advances in Rhinosinusitis and Nasal Polyposis, pp. 99-102
Edited by Hideyuki Kawauchi, Desiderio Passali, Ranko Mladina, Andrey Lopatin and Dmytro Zabolotnyi
2015 © Kugler Publications, Amsterdam, The Netherlands

player to this non-coding field and offer potentially new insights into the field of gene regulation.

The first few lncRNAs, of which XIST (X-inactive specific transcript) is a major example, were discovered in the 1990s by searching cDNA libraries for clones of interest, largely with the intention towards discovering new protein-coding genes.[7] Yet, in the last decade, there has been a shift in focus. The use of high-throughput technologies allows for a more unbiased approach to RNA discovery. Due to this shift in technology alone, the function of lncRNAs has slowly been able to be elucidated. XIST is a key player in X inactivation and exerts its function through such a recruitment of polycomb repressor complex 2 (PRC2), ultimately resulting in epigenetic silencing of one of the two human female X chromosomes.[7] Another well-characterized and early isolated lncRNAs is HOTAIR or HOX antisense intergenic RNA. Similar to XIST, HOTAIR works in an epigenetic fashion through the interaction of PRC2; it leads to the silencing of the HOXD locus, a key locus involved in limb patterning.[2] LncRNAs have also been found to be up regulated in response to various types of cellular stress. DNA damage can induce the expression of both lncRNA-p21 and PANDA, both of which are involved in regulating apoptosis.[8,9] The mechanism by which these lncRNAs regulate gene expression has been hypothesized and broadly classified to work as one of the following: signal, decoy, guide or scaffold.[10] A common theme in many of the lncRNAs ability to regulate gene expression involves their ability to recruit various chromatin-modifying complexes, such as EZH2 in PRC2 and CBX7 in PRC1.[11,12] However, more recently, a cytosolic acting lncRNA has been discovered, regulating its target genes through post-transcriptional mechanisms.[13] Since relatively little is still understood about lncRNAs, it will be interesting to see further developments beyond the predominantly nuclear, transcriptional mechanisms elucidated so far.

In addition to the role of lncRNAs in gene regulation, emerging evidence suggests that these non-coding RNAs may play a role in cancer biology. Abnormal expression of lncRNAs have been associated with a wide variety of cancers, most notably prostate and breast cancers. HOTAIR has been found to play an important role in breast cancer metastasis, with high expression of HOTAIR correlated to a more invasive phenotype leading to a higher likelihood of a poor outcome.[11] PCAT-1, Prostate Cancer Associated Transcript 1, is involved in prostate cancer cell proliferation and is thought to inhibit BRCA2, a known tumor suppressor gene.[14] Two lncRNAs, lncRNA-p21 and PANDA, are involved in p53 signaling and regulating the cellular response to DNA damage, can alter a cells response to chemotherapeutic drugs, such as doxorubicin.[8,9] Another lncRNA, GAS5, is down regulated in breast cancers and is thought to act like a tumor suppressor, arresting growth and promoting apoptosis in the cell.[15] Despite the known association of lncRNAs with cancer, the specific mechanisms by which these non-coding RNAs may affect various types of cancer behavior (carcinogenesis, drug resistance, metastasis, etc.) is still relatively unclear.

Lung cancer is the most prevalent cancer worldwide and is the leading cancer killer among all cancer types, accounting for 29% of all male deaths and 26%

of all female deaths here in the United States.[16] A strong link between cigarette smoking and lung cancer (specifically small cell and non-small cell lung cancers) has been well documented, with smoking contribution estimated to have been the key cause of 80 to 90% of all lung cancer deaths.[16] Although a well-established link has been shown, the molecular mechanism from smoke-induced epithelial cell injury that leads to lung cancer remains relatively unclear.

To date, only three long non-coding RNAs have been characterized to have a functional role in lung cancer: MALAT-1, emx2os and SCAL1. MALAT-1 or metastasis associated lung adenocarcinoma transcript 1, actively regulates gene expression of a variety of genes, including a set of genes involved in metastasis.[17] Further work has shown that MALAT1-deficient cells are impaired in migration and form fewer tumor nodules in a mouse xenograft model.[18] Emx2os, a type of antisense ncRNA, contributes to post-transcriptional down-regulation of its sense partner, EMX2, possibly in an epigenetic manner.[19] EMX2, empty spiracles gene 2, has been implicated as a tumor suppressor gene and its down-regulation is correlated with tumor progression in many types of cancer, including lung adenocarcinomas.[19] Our group has previously characterized SCAL1, Smoke and Cancer Associated LncRNA1, the first smoking-associated lncRNA.[20] We discovered this lncRNA by data mining publically available mRNA-seq datasets, comparing smokers to non-smokers. As a follow-up, we validated this target in our lab. SCAL1 was induced by cigarette smoke, both *in vitro* and *in vivo,* and elevated in various lung cancer cell lines.[20] We further demonstrated its expression was dependent upon NRF2 (nuclear factor erythroid 2-related factor 2) activation, via siRNA knockdown of NRF2 and KEAP1 resulting in a change in expression as well as a chromatin immunoprecipitation assay showing NRF2 binding to the SCAL1 promoter following cigarette smoke exposure.[20] Our previous publication identified a novel and interesting new non-coding RNA that may mediate some of the chemo resistance properties of NRF2 in lung cancer and may also provide a mechanistic link between cigarette smoking and lung cancer prognosis. We present our hypothesized model for how we believe SCAL1 promotes lung cancer formation in Figure 1.

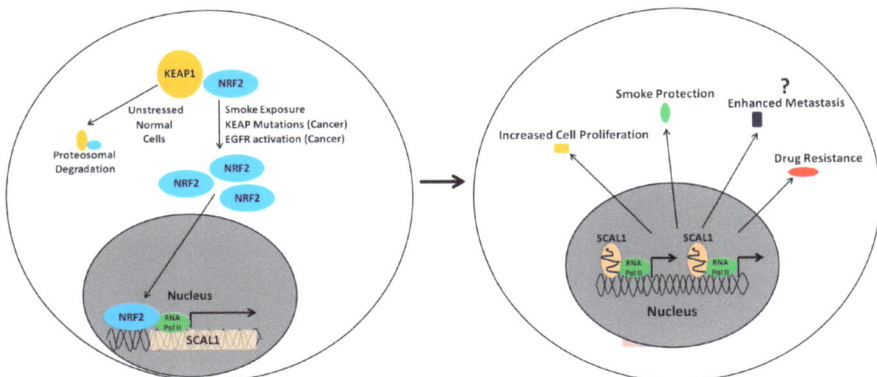

Fig. 1.   ■ author: please supply caption for this figure.

References

1. Birney E, Stamatoyannopoulos JA, Dutta A, et al. Identification and analysis of functional elements in 1% of the human genome by the ENCODE pilot project. Nature 2007;447(7146):799-816.
2. Rinn JL, Kertesz M, Wang JK, et al. Functional demarcation of active and silent chromatin domains in human HOX loci by noncoding RNAs. Cell 2007;129(7):1311-1323.
3. Taft RJ, Pang KC, Mercer TR, Dinger M, Mattick JS. Non-coding RNAs: regulators of disease. J Pathol 2010;220(2):126-139.
4. Moran VA, Perera RJ, Khalil AM. Emerging functional and mechanistic paradigms of mammalian long non-coding RNAs. Nucleic Acids Res 2012;40(14):6391-6400.
5. Guttman M, Amit I, Garber M, et al. Chromatin signature reveals over a thousand highly conserved large non-coding RNAs in mammals. Nature 2009;458(7235):223-227.
6. Pauli A, Rinn JL, Schier AF. Non-coding RNAs as regulators of embryogenesis. Nature Rev Gen 2011;12(2):136-149.
7. Plath K, Mlynarczyk-Evans S, Nusinow DA, Panning B. Xist RNA and the mechanism of X chromosome inactivation. Ann Rev Gen 2002;36:233-278.
8. Huarte M, Guttman M, Feldser D, et al. A large intergenic noncoding RNA induced by p53 mediates global gene repression in the p53 response. Cell 2010;142(3):409-419.
9. Hung T, Wang Y, Lin MF, et al. Extensive and coordinated transcription of noncoding RNAs within cell-cycle promoters. Nature Gen 2011;43(7):621-629.
10. Wang KC, Chang HY. Molecular mechanisms of long noncoding RNAs. Mol Cell 2011;43(6):904-914.
11. Gupta RA, Shah N, Wang KC, et al. Long non-coding RNA HOTAIR reprograms chromatin state to promote cancer metastasis. Nature 2010;464(7291):1071-1076.
12. Yap KL, Li S, Munoz-Cabello AM, et al. Molecular interplay of the noncoding RNA ANRIL and methylated histone H3 lysine 27 by polycomb CBX7 in transcriptional silencing of INK4a. Mol Cell 2010;38(5):662-674.
13. Carrieri C, Cimatti L, Biagioli M, et al. Long non-coding antisense RNA controls Uchl1 translation through an embedded SINEB2 repeat. Nature 2012;491(7424):454-457.
14. Prensner JR, Iyer MK, Balbin OA, et al. Transcriptome sequencing across a prostate cancer cohort identifies PCAT-1, an unannotated lincRNA implicated in disease progression. Nature Biotechnol 2011;29(8):742-749.
15. Mourtada-Maarabouni M, Pickard MR, Hedge VL, Farzaneh F, Williams GT. GAS5, a non-protein-coding RNA, controls apoptosis and is downregulated in breast cancer. Oncogene 2009;28(2):195-208.
16. ACS. Cancer Facts and Figures, 2012. http://tinyurl.com/7xcsdxg.
17. Ji P, Diederichs S, Wang W, et al. MALAT-1, a novel noncoding RNA, and thymosin beta4 predict metastasis and survival in early-stage non-small cell lung cancer. Oncogene 2003;22(39):8031-8041.
18. Tripathi V, Ellis JD, Shen Z, et al. The nuclear-retained noncoding RNA MALAT1 regulates alternative splicing by modulating SR splicing factor phosphorylation. Mol Cell 2010;39(6):925-938.
19. Okamoto J, Kratz JR, Hirata T, et al. Downregulation of EMX2 is associated with clinical outcomes in lung adenocarcinoma patients. Clin Lung Cancer 2011;12(4):237-244.
20. Thai P, Statt S, Chen CH, Liang E, Campbell C, Wu R. Characterization of a novel long noncoding RNA, SCAL1, induced by cigarette smoke and elevated in lung cancer cell lines. Amer J Resp Cell Mol Biol 2013;49(2): 204-211.

ROLE OF MUCINS IN RESPIRATORY TRACT INFLAMMATION

Kosuke Kato[1], Sheng Wang[1], Yong Lin[2], and K. Chul Kim[3]

[1]Center for Inflammation, Translational and Clinical Lung Research, Temple University School of Medicine, Philadelphia, PA 19140, USA; [2]Lovelace Respiratory Research Institute, Albuquerque, NM 87108, USA; [2]University of Arizona college of Medicine, Department of Otolaryngology, Tucson, AZ, USA

Abstract

Mucins are high molecular weight O-linked glycoproteins that are expressed in various mucosal epithelial cells as gel-forming, secreted or membrane-tethered forms. Twenty-two mucin genes have currently been identified in humans and 16 of them expressed in the lung. However, their roles are not fully understood. Based on their anatomical location, there is no doubt that they have an important defensive function. In fact, secreted mucins have been shown to be tightly associated with various biologically active molecules like 'aircraft carriers'. This section will provide a brief overview of our current understanding of the functions of the respiratory mucins in the context of lung physiology and pathology.

Introduction

Mucins are high molecular weight glycoproteins that are responsible for the viscoelastic property of the respiratory tract mucus. At least 22 mucin genes have been cloned in humans,[1-4] 16 of which have been identified in the respiratory tract ((MUC1, MUC2, MUC4, MUC5AC, MUC5B, MUC7, MUC8, MUC11, MUC13, MUC15, MUC16, MUC18, MUC19, MUC20, MUC21, and MUC22).[1,3-6] Deduced amino acid sequences of the cloned mucin genes revealed that there are two types of mucins – secreted mucins and membrane-tethered mucins. Seven

Address for correspondence: Dr. Kwang Chul Kim, University of Arizona college of Medicine, Department of Otolaryngology Tucson, AZ 85724, USA.
E-mail:Kckim@oto.arizona.edu

Recent Advances in Rhinosinusitis and Nasal Polyposis, pp. 103-109
Edited by Hideyuki Kawauchi, Desiderio Passali, Ranko Mladina, Andrey Lopatin
and Dmytro Zabolotnyi
2015 © Kugler Publications, Amsterdam, The Netherlands

mucin gene products (*i.e.*, MUC2, 5AC, 5B, 6, 7, 8 and 19) are characterized as secreted and the remaining ten mucin gene products are membrane-tethered.[4,7] Most of the transmembrane mucins are found on the apical surface of lining mucosal epithelial cells that are in contact with the outside environment, suggesting a defensive role of these epithelial mucins for the host.

Mucins as a scaffold protein

Based on its anatomical location in the body as well as the complex structure of mucins, it was suggested quite some time ago that mucus has multifaceted properties necessary for host defense: anti-microbial, anti-protease, and anti-oxidant activities. Jacquot *et al.*[8] first reported the presence of these properties in airway secretions. Kim *et al.*[9,10] demonstrated that airway mucins are extremely hydrophobic and even guanidine hydrochloride (4-6 M), one of the most chaotrophic agents, could not completely dissociate mucins from other macromolecules present in airway secretion. It was postulated that the hydrophobic property may allow for efficient packaging of these highly thermodynamic mucins ($> 10^6$ Dalton) into the distinct secretory granules.[11] Recent proteomics analysis of mucins revealed that mucins are tightly associated with various proteins,[12,13] including those with anti-microbial, anti-protease, anti-oxidant, or anti-inflammatory properties.[13] Thus, mucins are like a large aircraft carrier carrying a variety of 'weapons' to be used against the invading pathogens. It may be possible that association of mucins with the bioactive molecules are formed inside the secretory granules before but not after exocytosis as previously suggested,[10] such that they can interact with invading pathogens more effectively and efficiently upon exocytosis. How and when such association takes place in the goblet cell and is packaged into a mucous granule remains to be uncovered.

Roles of muciins in the respiratory tract

Although 16 out of 22 mucin genes (MUC in human and Muc in nonhuman species) have been identified in the lung, their functions are largely unknown. A recent review by Sheehan *et al.*[14] describes the roles of five major mucns (MUC5AC, MUC5B, MUC1, MUC4, and MUC16) in protecting and stabilizing the ciliated surface and building the gel in the airway epithelium. The roles of these mucins were also reviewed by Kim[15] with a focus on the anti-inflammatory role of MUC1 during airway infection. In this presentation, we will update our knowledge of the roles of these mucins in the lung.

Membrane-tethered mucins (MUC1, MUC4 and MUC16)

MUC1 is the first mucin gene cloned[16,17] as a cancer antigen. In the lung, MUC1 has been shown to be expressed in airway[18-20] and alveolar type II[21] epithelial cells, dendritic cells[22] and monocytes/macrophages.[23] It plays an anti-inflammatory role during bacterial infection of the lung based on animal experiments.[24-27] Detailed mechanistic studies with airway epithelial cells revealed that TNF-a produced during inflammation upregulates MUC1[25,28] which is then tyrosine-phosphorylated by EGFR that is also activated by TGF-a during inflammation.[29] Phosphorylated MUC1 then binds to Toll-like receptors (TLRs) preventing the recruitment of either MyD88[29] or TRIF[30] to their corresponding TLRs, which results in suppression of TLR signaling. Interestingly, the suppression of TLR signaling by MUC1 seems to be applicable to all TLRs[31] thus making MUC1 a universal inhibitor of TLR signaling. Given the importance of host defense during infection, one may wonder if the anti-inflammatory activity of MUC1 could be detrimental to the host. However, MUC1 is upregulated by a major pro-inflammatory agent (i.e., TNF-a) during infection to control inflammation thus forming a feedback loop of inflammation. In fact, mice deficient in Muc1 showed excessive lung inflammation and injuries following bacterial infection in both acute[25] and chronic[26] *Pseudomonas aeruginosa* infection models. The anti-inflammatory effects of MUC1 was also demonstrated in dendritic cells *in vitro*[32] as well as in an animal model of autoimmune disease.[33] It is of note that all these mechanistic studies have been carried out exclusively in airway epithelial cells. Whether MUC1 has the same role in other lung cell types such as alveolar type II cells and macrophages remains unknown and certainly an important area to explore in order to fully understand the roles of MUC1 during the respiratory infection and inflammation.

In addition to MUC1, both MUC4 and MUC16 have been shown to be produced and released by airway surface epithelial cells.[12] Sheehan et al.[14] demonstrated that shed mucins form a gel in the immediate vicinity of the apical cell surface, likely serving as a protective barrier against invading pathogens and chemicals. How and when these membrane glycoproteins are cleaved remains largely unknown and will be important questions to address in the context with respiratory tract infection and inflammation.

Gel-forming mucins (MUC5AC and MUC5B)

Four major gel-forming mucins have been reported to be present in the lung – MUC2, MUC5AC, MUC5B and MUC19. Although MUC2 was shown to be associated with cystic fibrosis[34] as well as bacterial infection,[35] its total absence in either normal or pathologic human sputum samples[36,37] seems to suggest that MUC2 is not a major mucin produced in the lung. MUC19, the major salivary glandular mucin,[38] has also been identified in tracheolarynx.[39] However, its role in the lung is totally unknown.

On the other hand, MUC5AC and MUC5B are the major gel-forming mucins in the airway and thus believed to contribute to both the defensive barrier function and the rheology of airway mucus. MUC5AC has been shown to be the goblet cell mucin,[40] whereas MUC5B has been shown to be the submucosal gland mucin.[41] MUC5AC has been widely used as a marker for goblet cell metaplasia[42] and has been shown to be associated with asthma.[43-45] Recent studies, however, have demonstrated that MUC5B is the major type of mucin produced by goblet cells[37] and associated with COPD.[46,47] It has been suggested that MUC5AC expression is inducible during airway inflammation,[43] whereas MUC5B expression is constitutive.[43,48] Interestingly, transgenic mice overexpressing MUC5AC demonstrated the normal mucus transport and absence of a pulmonary phenotype suggesting that MUC5AC hypersecretion alone is not sufficient to trigger luminal mucus plugging or airways inflammation/goblet cell hyperplasia.[49] However, these mice exhibited a protective role against influenza infection. On the other hand, mice deficient in MUC5B showed impaired mucociliary clearance leading to bacterial infection in airways, whereas MUC5AC was dispensable.[47] Interestingly, a MUC5B promoter polymorphism has been associated with pulmonary fibrosis.[50,51] Airway disease associated with mucus dysfunction has recently been reviewed.[52]

Conclusion

Airway surface fluid contains two layers of mucins consisting mainly of five different mucin gene products. While the outer layer contains mainly two gel-forming mucins (MUC5AC and MUC5B) that are tightly associated with various biologically active, defensive molecules, the inner layer contains three membrane-tethered mucins (MUC1, MUC4 and MUC16) shed from the apical cell surface. During airway infection, all of these mucins serve as a major protective barrier against pathogens. MUC1 mucin produced by virtually all the surface columnar epithelial cells in the respiratory tract as well as Type II pneumocytes in the alveoli plays an additional, perhaps more critical role during respiratory infection by controlling the resolution of inflammation to prevent the development of inflammatory lung disease. The current availability of genetically modified mice in these mucin genes will undoubtedly expedite the research toward our better understanding of the roles of respiratory mucins in physiology and pathology and eventually contribute to the diagnosis, prevention and treatment of various respiratory inflammatory diseases.

References

1. Rose MC, Voynow JA. Respiratory tract mucin genes and mucin glycoproteins in health and disease. Physiol Rev 2006;86(1):245-278. doi: 10.1152/physrev.00010.2005.
2. Yi Y, Kamata-Sakurai M, Denda-Nagai K, et al. Mucin 21/epiglycanin modulates cell adhesion. J Biol Chem 2010;285(28):21233-21240. doi: 10.1074/jbc.M109.082875.
3. Itoh Y, Kamata-Sakurai M, Denda-Nagai K, et al. Identification and expression of human epiglycanin/MUC21: A novel transmembrane mucin. Glycobiology 2008;18(1):74-83. doi: 10.1093/glycob/cwm118.
4. Hijikata M, Matsushita I, Tanaka G, et al. Molecular cloning of two novel mucin-like genes in the disease-susceptibility locus for diffuse panbronchiolitis. Hum Genet 2011;129(2):117-128. doi: 10.1007/s00439-010-0906-4.

5. Davies JR, Kirkham S, Svitacheva N, Thornton DJ, Carlstedt I. MUC16 is produced in tracheal surface epithelium and submucosal glands and is present in secretions from normal human airway and cultured bronchial epithelial cells. Int J Biochem Cell Biol 2007;39(10):1943-1954. doi: 10.1016/j.biocel.2007.05.013.

6. Simon GC, Martin RJ, Smith S, et al. Up-regulation of MUC18 in airway epithelial cells by IL-13: Implications in bacterial adherence. Am J Respir Cell Mol Biol 2011;44(5):606-613. doi: 10.1165/rcmb.2010-0384OC.

7. Thornton DJ, Rousseau K, McGuckin MA. Structure and function of the polymeric mucins in airways mucus. Annu Rev Physiol 2008;70:459-486. doi: 10.1146/annurev.physiol.70.113006.100702.

8. Jacquot J, Hayem A, Galabert C. Functions of proteins and lipids in airway secretions. Eur Respir J 1992;5(3):343-358.

9. Kim KC, Opaskar-Hincman H, Bhaskar KR. Secretions from primary hamster tracheal surface epithelial cells in culture: Mucin-like glycoproteins, proteoglycans, and lipids. Exp Lung Res 1989;15(2):299-314.

10. Kim KC, Singh BN. Association of lipids with mucins may take place prior to secretion: Studies with primary hamster tracheal epithelial cells in culture. Biorheology 1990;27(3-4):491-501.

11. Kim KC. Regulation of airway goblet cell mucin secretion. In: T. Takishima, S. Shimura (Eds.), Airway secretion: Physiological bases for the control of mucus hypersecretion. Lung biology and health vol. 72, pp. 433-449. New York, NY: Marcel Dekker, Inc. 1993.

12. Kesimer M, Scull M, Brighton B, et al. Characterization of exosome-like vesicles released from human tracheobronchial ciliated epithelium: A possible role in innate defense. FASEB J 2009;23(6):1858-1868. doi: 10.1096/fj.08-119131.

13. Ali M, Lillehoj EP, Park Y, Kyo Y, Kim KC. Analysis of the proteome of human airway epithelial secretions. Proteome Sci 2011;9:4. doi: 10.1186/1477-5956-9-4.

14. Sheehan JK, Kesimer M, Pickles R. Innate immunity and mucus structure and function. Novartis Found Symp 2006;279:155-66; discussion 167-169, 216-219.

15. Kim KC. Role of epithelial mucins during airway infection. Pulm Pharmacol Ther 2012;25(6):415-419. doi: 10.1016/j.pupt.2011.12.003.

16. Gendler SJ, Lancaster CA, Taylor-Papadimitriou J, et al. Molecular cloning and expression of human tumor-associated polymorphic epithelial mucin. J Biol Chem 1990;265(25):15286-15293.

17. Lan MS, Batra SK, Qi WN, Metzgar RS, Hollingsworth MA. Cloning and sequencing of a human pancreatic tumor mucin cDNA. J Biol Chem 1990;265(25):15294-15299.

18. Pemberton L, Taylor-Papadimitriou J, Gendler SJ. Antibodies to the cytoplasmic domain of the MUC1 mucin show conservation throughout mammals. Biochem Biophys Res Commun 1992;185(1):167-175.

19. Hollingsworth MA, Batra SK, Qi WN, Yankaskas JR. MUC1 mucin mRNA expression in cultured human nasal and bronchial epithelial cells. Am J Respir Cell Mol Biol 1992;6(5):516-520.

20. Park H, Hyun SW, Kim KC. Expression of MUC1 mucin gene by hamster tracheal surface epithelial cells in primary culture. Am J Respir Cell Mol Biol 1996;15(2):237-244.

21. Kohno N, Kyoizumi S, Awaya Y, et al. New serum indicator of interstitial pneumonitis activity. sialylated carbohydrate antigen KL-6. Chest 1989;96(1):68-73.

22. Wykes M, MacDonald KP, Tran M, et al. MUC1 epithelial mucin (CD227) is expressed by activated dendritic cells. J Leukoc Biol 2002;72(4):692-701.

23. Leong CF, Raudhawati O, Cheong SK, et al. Epithelial membrane antigen (EMA) or MUC1 expression in monocytes and monoblasts. Pathology 2003;35(5):422-427. doi: N2B2VP3K-46WE6QM2 [pii].

24. Lu W, Hisatsune A, Koga T, et al. Cutting edge: Enhanced pulmonary clearance of pseudomonas aeruginosa by Muc1 knockout mice. J Immunol 2006;176(7):3890-3894.

25. Choi S, Park YS, Koga T, Treloar A, Kim KC. TNF-alpha is a key regulator of MUC1, an anti-inflammatory molecule, during airway pseudomonas aeruginosa infection. Am J Respir Cell Mol Biol 2011;44(2):255-260. doi: 10.1165/rcmb.2009-0323OC.

26. Umehara T, Kato K, Park YS, et al. Prevention of lung injury by Muc1 mucin in a mouse model of repetitive pseudomonas aeruginosa infection. Inflamm Res 2012;61(9):1013-1020. doi: 10.1007/s00011-012-0494-y.

27. Kim KC, Lillehoj EP. MUC1 mucin: A peacemaker in the lung. Am J Respir Cell Mol Biol 2008;39(6):644-647. doi: 10.1165/rcmb.2008-0169TR.

28. Koga T, Kuwahara I, Lillehoj EP, et al. TNF-alpha induces MUC1 gene transcription in lung epithelial cells: Its signaling pathway and biological implication. Am J Physiol Lung Cell Mol Physiol 2007;293(3):L693-701. doi: 10.1152/ajplung.00491.2006.

29. Kato K, Lillehoj EP, Park YS, et al. Membrane-tethered MUC1 mucin is phosphorylated by epidermal growth factor receptor in airway epithelial cells and associates with TLR5 to inhibit recruitment of MyD88. J Immunol 2012;188:2014-2022. doi: 10.4049/jimmunol.1102405.

30. Kato K, Lillehoj EP, Kim KC. MUC1 regulates epithelial inflammation and apoptosis by PolyI:C through inhibition of TRIF recruitment to TLR3. Am J Respir Cell Mol Biol 2014. doi: 10.1165/rcmb.2014-0018OC [doi].

31. Ueno K, Koga T, Kato K, et al. MUC1 mucin is a negative regulator of toll-like receptor signaling. Am J Respir Cell Mol Biol 2008;38(3):263-268. doi: 10.1165/rcmb.2007-0336RC.

32. Williams MA, Bauer S, Lu W, et al. Deletion of the mucin-like molecule muc1 enhances dendritic cell activation in response to toll-like receptor ligands. J Innate Immun 2010;2(2):123-143. doi: 10.1159/000254790.

33. Yen JH, Xu S, Park YS, Ganea D, Kim KC. Higher susceptibility to experimental autoimmune encephalomyelitis in Muc1-deficient mice is associated with increased Th1/Th17 responses. Brain Behav Immun 2013;29:70-81. doi: 10.1016/j.bbi.2012.12.004 [doi].

34. Li JD, Dohrman AF, Gallup M, et al. Transcriptional activation of mucin by pseudomonas aeruginosa lipopolysaccharide in the pathogenesis of cystic fibrosis lung disease. Proc Natl Acad Sci U S A 1997;94(3):967-972.

35. Dohrman A, Miyata S, Gallup M, et al. Mucin gene (MUC 2 and MUC 5AC) upregulation by gram-positive and gram-negative bacteria. Biochim Biophys Acta 1998;1406(3):251-259.

36. Hovenberg HW, Davies JR, Herrmann A, Linden CJ, Carlstedt I. MUC5AC, but not MUC2, is a prominent mucin in respiratory secretions. Glycoconj J 1996;13(5):839-847.

37. Kesimer M, Kirkham S, Pickles RJ, et al. Tracheobronchial air-liquid interface cell culture: A model for innate mucosal defense of the upper airways? Am J Physiol Lung Cell Mol Physiol 2009;296(1):L92-L100. doi: 10.1152/ajplung.90388.2008.

38. Chen Y, Zhao YH, Kalaslavadi TB, et al. Genome-wide search and identification of a novel gel-forming mucin MUC19/Muc19 in glandular tissues. Am J Respir Cell Mol Biol 2004;30(2):155-165. doi: 10.1165/rcmb.2003-0103OC.

39. Das B, Cash MN, Hand AR, et al. Tissue distibution of murine Muc19/smgc gene products. J Histochem Cytochem 2009. doi: 10.1369/jhc.2009.954891.

40. Hovenberg HW, Davies JR, Carlstedt I. Different mucins are produced by the surface epithelium and the submucosa in human trachea: Identification of MUC5AC as a major mucin from the goblet cells. Biochem J 1996;318 (Pt 1)(Pt 1):319-324.

41. Wickstrom C, Davies JR, Eriksen GV, Veerman EC, Carlstedt I. MUC5B is a major gel-forming, oligomeric mucin from human salivary gland, respiratory tract and endocervix: Identification of glycoforms and C-terminal cleavage. Biochem J 1998;334 (Pt 3)(Pt 3):685-693.

42. Zuhdi Alimam M, Piazza FM, Selby DM, et al. Muc-5/5ac mucin messenger RNA and protein expression is a marker of goblet cell metaplasia in murine airways. Am J Respir Cell Mol Biol 2000;22(3):253-260.

43. Evans CM, Kim K, Tuvim MJ, Dickey BF. Mucus hypersecretion in asthma: Causes and effects. Curr Opin Pulm Med 2009;15(1):4-11. doi: 10.1097/MCP.0b013e32831da8d3.

44. Ordonez CL, Khashayar R, Wong HH, et al. Mild and moderate asthma is associated with airway goblet cell hyperplasia and abnormalities in mucin gene expression. Am J Respir Crit Care Med 2001;163(2):517-523.

45. Hallstrand TS, Debley JS, Farin FM, Henderson WR, Jr. Role of MUC5AC in the pathogenesis of exercise-induced bronchoconstriction. J Allergy Clin Immunol 2007;119(5):1092-1098. doi: 10.1016/j.jaci.2007.01.005.

46. Kirkham S, Kolsum U, Rousseau K, et al. MUC5B is the major mucin in the gel phase of sputum in chronic obstructive pulmonary disease. Am J Respir Crit Care Med 2008;178(10):1033-1039. doi: 10.1164/rccm.200803-391OC.

47. Roy MG, Livraghi-Butrico A, Fletcher AA, et al. Muc5b is required for airway defence. Nature. 2014;505(7483):412-416. doi: 10.1038/nature12807 [doi].

48. Roy MG, Rahmani M, Hernandez JR, et al. Mucin production during pre- and post-natal mouse lung development. Am J Respir Cell Mol Biol 2011. doi: 10.1165/rcmb.2010-0020RC.

49. Ehre C, Worthington EN, Liesman RM, et al. Overexpressing mouse model demonstrates the protective role of Muc5ac in the lungs. Proc Natl Acad Sci U S A 2012;109(41):16528-16533. doi: 10.1073/pnas.1206552109 [doi].

50. Seibold MA, Wise AL, Speer MC, et al. A common MUC5B promoter polymorphism and pulmonary fibrosis. N Engl J Med 2011;364(16):1503-1512. doi: 10.1056/NEJMoa1013660.

51. Steele MP, Schwartz DA. Molecular mechanisms in progressive idiopathic pulmonary fibrosis. Annu Rev Med 2013;64:265-276. doi: 10.1146/annurev-med-042711-142004 [doi].

52. Fahy JV, Dickey BF. Airway mucus function and dysfunction. N Engl J Med 2010;363(23):2233-2247. doi: 10.1056/NEJMra0910061.

ROLE OF COAGULATION FACTORS AND EOSINOPHILS IN THE PATHOGENESIS OF MUCUS HYPERSECRETION IN EOSINOPHIL-ASSOCIATED CHRONIC RHINOSINUSITIS

Takeshi Shimizu, Shino Shimizu, Takao Ogawa, Kumiko Takezawa, Hideaki Kouzaki

Department of Otorhinolaryngology, Shiga University of Medical Science, Otsu, Japan

Introduction

Eosinophil-associated chronic rhinosinusitis (CRS) is characterized by predominant eosinophil infiltration, hypersecretion of sticky and glue-like mucus, and tissue remodeling such as goblet cell metaplasia, hyperplasia of nasal mucosal cells and formation of nasal polyps. Several cytokines, chemokines and growth factors are involved in the pathogenesis of mucus hypersecretion and airway tissue remodeling. MUC5AC mucin is predominant in airway inflammation and is up regulated in nasal polyposis.[1] Platelet-derived growth factor (PDGF) and vascular endothelial growth factor (VEGF) are important cytokines with a crucial role in tissue remodeling. PDGF stimulates growth of fibroblast and production of extracellular matrix. VEGF increases vascular permeability and stimulates the proliferation of vascular endothelial cells. PDGF and VEGF have been reported to play a role in the formation of nasal polyps in CRS patients.[2,3]

We found numerous fibrin depositions in sticky mucus and subepithelial tissues of nasal polyps from patients with eosinophil-associated CRS, indicating that the coagulation system is locally activated in nasal mucus and tissues. Eosinophils are the principal effector cells in nasal polyposis and bronchial asthma. There is increasing evidences indicating that eosinophil-epithelial cell interactions are crucial in the initiation and development of airway inflamma-

Address for correspondence: Takeshi Shimizu MD, Department of Otorhinolaryngology. Shiga University of Medical Science. Seta-Tsukinowa, Otsu, Shiga 520-2192, Japan. Tel: +81-77-548-2261. Fax: +81-77-548-2783. E-mail: shimizu@belle.shiga-md.ac.jp

Recent Advances in Rhinosinusitis and Nasal Polyposis, pp. 111-116
Edited by Hideyuki Kawauchi, Desiderio Passali, Ranko Mladina, Andrey Lopatin and Dmytro Zabolotnyi
2015 © Kugler Publications, Amsterdam, The Netherlands

tion. We hypothesized that coagulation factors and eosinophil-epithelial cell interactions are involved in the pathogenesis of mucus hypersecretion and tissue remodeling in eosinophil-associated CRS.

Thrombin is the effector enzyme of the coagulation system with important biological functions not only in thrombosis and hemostasis, but also in inflammation through protease activated receptor (PAR)-1, -3 and -4. Firstly, in the present study, to elucidate the role of coagulation factors in mucus hypersecretion and tissue remodeling, we measured the concentrations of thrombin and thrombin-antithrombin (TAT) complex in nasal secretion from CRS patients, and examined the effects of thrombin or PAR-1 agonist peptide on the secretions of MUC5AC mucin, PDGF and VEGF from cultured human airway epithelial cells.[3-5] The effect of intranasal instillation with thrombin was examined in rat nasal epithelium.[4] Secondly, to elucidate the role of eosinophil-epithelial cell interactions, the productions of MUC5AC mucin, PDGF and VEGF were examined in human airway epithelial (NCI-H292) cells co-cultured with human eosinophilic (EoL-1) cells or with human blood eosinophils.[6]

Methods

Nasal secretion was collected from patients with chronic rhinosinusitis with nasal polyp (CRSwNP) with asthma (n = 9), CRSwNP without asthma (n = 10), allergic rhinitis (AR) (n = 7), and control patients (n = 3). The concentrations of thrombin, thrombin-antithrombin (TAT) complex, MUC5AC mucin, platelet-derived growth factor (PDGF) and vascular endothelial growth factor (VEGF) were evaluated by enzyme immunoassays. The mRNA expressions of MUC5AC mucin, PDGF, VEGF and PAR-1 were examined by reverse transcription-polymerase chain reaction (RT-PCR). Tissue localization of thrombin receptor (PAR-1) and tissue factor (an important initial upstream protein in extrinsic coagulation pathway) were immunohistochemically studied in nasal epithelium. The concentrations of thrombin and TAT complex were measured in nasal secretion from each group of patients.[4] The concentrations of MUC5AC mucin, PDGF and VEGF were measured in culture medium from airway epithelial cells treated with thrombin or thrombin receptor (PAR-1) agonist peptide.[3-5] The effect of intranasal instillation with thrombin was histologically examined in the nasal epithelium of F344 rats (eight to ten weeks of age).[4]

The human airway epithelial (NCI-H292) cells were plated on six-well or 24-well culture plates. After confluent cells were cultured in RPMI-1640 for 18 h, and then were co-cultured with human eosinophilic (EoL-1) cells or with human blood eosinophils for 24 h. Conditioned medium was harvested, and total RNA was collected from NCI-H292 cells and EoL-1 cells separately. Productions of MUC5AC mucin, PDGF and VEGF were examined.[6]

Results

Coagulation activation markers in nasal secretion

Significant concentrations of thrombin and TAT complex were found in nasal secretion, and they were significantly elevated in nasal secretion from patients with AR and CRSwNP with asthma compared to the control group.[2] Tissue factor is an initial upstream protein in extrinsic coagulation cascade, and was immunohistochemically localized in the epithelial cells and infiltrating cells of nasal polyps. Tissue factor activity was determined as factor X activation by factor VIIa/tissue factor complex, and thrombin or tumor necrosis factor (TNF)-α enhanced tissue factor activity of the surface of cultured epithelial (A549) cells.[3,4] These results indicate that airway inflammation enhances the activation of coagulation system, and it may be involved in the pathogenesis of eosinophil-associated CRS.

In-vitro effects of thrombin on secretions of MUC5AC mucin, PDGF and VEGF

We confirmed that thrombin receptor, PAR-1 was immunohistochemically localized in the epithelial cells of nasal polyps. Thrombin (62.5-500 nM) or PAR-1 agonist peptide (25-100 μM) significantly stimulated the secretions of MUC5AC mucin, VEGF and PDGF from cultured normal human bronchial epithelial (NHBE) cells or from nasal epithelial cells cultured at air-liquid interface in a dose-dependent manner. These results indicate that the effects of thrombin on secretions of MUC5AC, PDGF and VEGF are mediated through PAR-1 receptor of epithelial cells. Thrombin-induced MUC5AC secretion was significantly inhibited by epidermal growth factor receptor (EGFR) tyrosine kinase inhibitor AG1478, and we confirmed that EGFR was immunohistochemically expressed in the epithelial cells of nasal polyps.[3-5] These results indicate that thrombin-induced EGFR transactivation may be involved in thrombin-induced MUC5AC secretion.

In-vivo effect of intranasal instillation with thrombin in rat nasal epithelium

Thrombin (20 μM) was instilled into both nasal cavities of F344 rats each day for three days. Hypertrophic changes of goblet cells and significant mucus production were induced in rat nasal epithelium at 24 h after the last intranasal instillation.[4]

Co-culture-induced productions of MUC5AC mucin and cytokines

The co-culture with EoL-1 cells for 24 hours significantly stimulated secretions of MUC5AC mucin, PDGF, VEGF, TGF-α and IL-8 from cultured epithelial (NCI-H292) cells depending on the numbers of EoL-1 cells. MUC5AC mRNA expression in NCI-H292 cells was increased by co-culture with EoL-1 cells for six hours. Co-culture with peripheral blood eosinophils also stimulated MU-C5AC secretion. Unstimulated EoL-1 cells did not secrete MUC5AC mucin and these cytokines. Co-culture-induced MUC5AC secretion was not inhibited by blocking the cell-to-cell contact between epithelial cells and EoL-1 cells using nylon mesh insert. However, the conditioned medium from EoL-1 cells did not stimulate MUC5AC secretion from epithelial cells.[6] These results indicate that the intercellular interactions between eosinophils and epithelial cells, but not the cell-to-cell contact are important for co-culture-induced MUC5AC secretion.

EGFR transactivation is important in co-culture-induced MUC5AC secretion

Co-culture-induced secretions of MUC5AC mucin, PDGF, VEGF and IL-8 were significantly inhibited by EGFR tyrosine kinase inhibitor AG1478. Neutralizing antibody against amphiregulin or TGF-α significantly inhibited co-culture-induced MUC5AC secretion. A broad-spectrum metalloproteinase inhibitor GM6001 significantly inhibited co-culture-induced secretions of MUC5AC, PDGF, VEGF and amphiregulin.[6] These results indicate that metalloproteinase-mediated, amphiregulin and TGF-α-induced EGFR transactivation may be important for co-culture-induced MUC5AC secretion (Fig. 1).

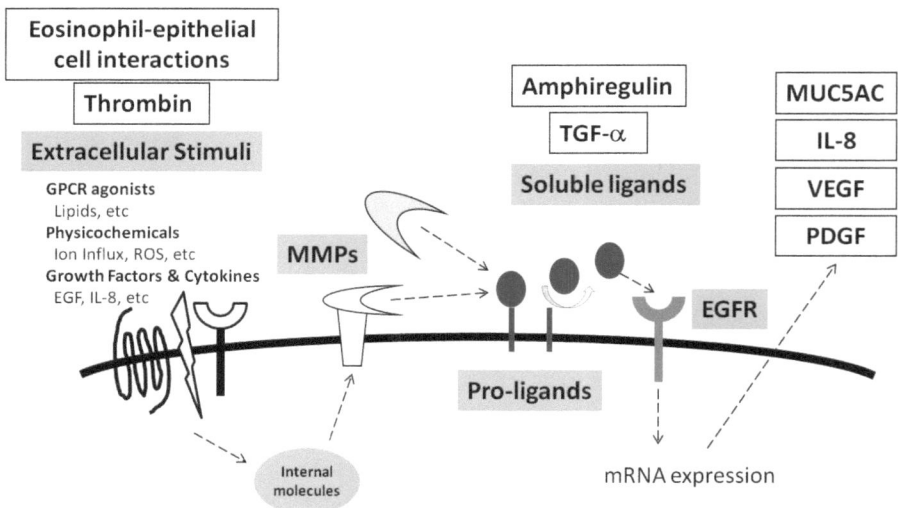

Fig. 1. A mechanism of ligand-shedding dependent EGFR transactivation. A membrane-anchored disintegrin and metalloproteinases (ADAMS), and cleaved pro-ligands such as TGF-a and amphiregulin are important in this process. Thrombin-induced MUC5AC secretion and eosinophil-epithelial cell interactions-induced secretions of MUC5AC, PDGF and VEGF are mediated through EGFR transactivation.

Discussion

The present study showed that significant local activation of the coagulation system with increased thrombin generation is involved in the pathogenesis of eosinophil-associated CRS and that thrombin promotes mucus hypersecretion and tissue remodeling by stimulating the secretions of MUC5AC mucin, PDGF and VEGF from airway epithelial cells via its receptor PAR-1. Thrombin is also important for tissue remodeling by enhancing fibrin deposition and by stimulating cell proliferation and extracellular matrix production of fibroblast and vascular endothelial cells. Because the activation of coagulation is important in the pathogenesis of CRS, the inhibition of coagulation factors may be a potential therapeutic target for the treatment of CRS patients. We found that intranasal instillation with anticoagulant drugs, heparin or activated protein C, attenuated airway inflammation such as goblet cell metaplasia and neutrophil infiltration in rat nasal epithelium by the inhibition of coagulation system and by the direct inhibitory effects on the secretions of MUC5AC mucin and IL-8 from airway epithelial cells.[4,7-9]

The present study also showed that eosinophil-epithelial cell interactions induce the secretions of MUC5AC mucin, PDGF and VEGF, which are important in the pathogenesis of mucus hypersecretion and tissue remodeling of eosinophil-predominant airway inflammation such as nasal polyposis and bronchial asthma. Metalloprotease-mediated EGFR transactivation plays a crucial role in eosinophil-epithelial cell interactions, and it is also involved in the thrombin-induced MUC5AC secretion (Fig. 1). EGFR signaling may be a potential therapeutic target for the treatment of CRS patients, and we found that the EGFR inhibitor attenuated LPS-induced mucus hypersecretion and neutrophil infiltration in rat nasal epithelium (data not shown).

In conclusion, activation of the coagulation system with increased thrombin generation and fibrin deposition is involved in the pathogenesis of mucus hypersecretion and tissue remodeling in eosinophil-associated CRS. Thrombin and eosinophil-epithelial cell interactions stimulate mucus hypersecretion from airway epithelial cells mediated by the EGFR transactivation. Anticoagulant drugs or EGFR inhibitor are potential therapeutic targets for the treatment of eosinophil-associated CRS.

References

1. Shimizu T. Mucus, goblet cell, submucosal gland. In: Önerci YM (Ed.), Nasal Physiology and pathophysiology of nasal disorders, pp. 1-14. Heidelberg: Springer 2013.
2. Kouzaki H, Seno S, Fukui J, Owaki S, Shimizu T. Role of platelet-derived growth factor in airway remodeling in rhinosinusitis. Am J Rhinol Allergy 2009;23:273-280.
3. Shimizu S, Gabazza EC, Ogawa T, et al. Role of thrombin in chronic rhinosinusitis-associated tissue remodeling. Am J Rhinol Allergy 2011;25;7-11.
4. Shimizu S, Shimizu T, Morser J, et al. Role of the coagulation system in allergic inflammation in the upper airways. Clin Immunol 2008;129;365-371.

5. Shimizu S, Gabazza EC, Hayashi T, et al. Thrombin stimulates the expression of PDGF in lung epithelial cells. Am J Physiol Lung Cell Mol Physiol 2001;279:L503-10.
6. Shimizu S, Kouzaki H, Shimizu T. Eosinophil-epithelial cell interactions stimulate the productions of MUC5AC mucin and profibrotic cytokines involved in airway tissue remodeling. Am J Rhinol Allergy 2014;28:103-109.
7. Ogawa T, Shimizu S, Tojima I, Kouzaki H, Shimizu T. Heparin inhibits mucus hypersecretion in airway epithelial cells. Am J Rhinol Allergy 2011;25;69-74.
8. Ogawa T, Shimizu S, Shimizu T. The effect of heparin on antigen-induced mucus hypersecretion in the nasal epithelium of sensitized rats. Allergol Int 2013;62:77-83.
9. Shimizu S, Gabazza EC, Taguchi O, et al. Activated protein C inhibits the expression of platelet-derived growth factor in the lung. Am J Respir Crit Care Med 2003;167:1416-1426.

PHARMACODYNAMICS OF ANTI-INFLAMMATORY DRUGS – INTRANASAL CORTICOSTEROID AND DNA DAMAGE

Yusuke Suzuki[1], Nobuo Ohta[1], Yuichi Takahashi[1], Shinpei Shibata[2], Seiji Kakehata[1], Yoshitaka Okamoto[3]

[1]Department of Otolaryngology, Head and Neck Surgery, Faculty of Medicine, Yamagata University, Yamagata, Japan; [2]Department of Physics, Faculty of Science, Yamagata University, Yamagata, Japan; [3]Department of Otolaryngology, Head and Neck Surgery, Graduate School of Medicine, Chiba University, Chiba, Japan

Abstract

Background: We examined the effect of intranasal corticosteroid on DNA damage in nasal smear cells from patients with allergic rhinitis, chronic rhinosinusitis and hyposmia. The effect of dexamethasone (DEX) on the DNA damage of healthy human peripheral blood lymphocytes (PBL) was also examined. **Methods:** Forty-eight patients with allergic rhinitis, 19 patients with chronic rhinitis and nine patients with hyposmia were enrolled in this study. A nasal smear was collected from each patient and the degree of DNA damage was evaluated by comet assay. PBL were incubated with DEX prior to UV-C irradiation. The DNA damage was introduced by 254 nm of 15 mJ/cm^2 UV-C and evaluated by single-cell microgel electrophoresis (Comet assay) under alkaline condition. **Results:** The infiltrating cells of the patients who used intranasal corticsteroids showed a lower proportion of damaged cells than those of the patients who used antihistamine drugs or leukotriene antagonists. The DNA damages of PBL were decreased by treatment with DEX in dose and time-dependent manner. **Conclusion:** Intranasal corticosteroid suppressed the DNA damage in nasal smear compared with other treatment modalities. Comet assay is a simple, easy and useful method to elucidate the mechanisms of intranasal corticosteroid.

Address for correspondence: Nobuo Ohta MD, Department of Otolaryngology, Head and Neck Surgery, Yamagata University Faculty of Medicine, 2-2-2 Iida-nishi, Yamagata 990-9585, Japan. E-mail: noohta@med.id.yamagata-u.ac.jp

Recent Advances in Rhinosinusitis and Nasal Polyposis, pp. 117-126
Edited by Hideyuki Kawauchi, Desiderio Passali, Ranko Mladina, Andrey Lopatin and Dmytro Zabolotnyi
2015 © Kugler Publications, Amsterdam, The Netherlands

Introduction

Inflammation is an important phenomenon in allergic disorders and intranasal corticosteroid drugs due to their anti-inflammatory properties have a pivotal role in improvement, control and relieving the symptoms and signs of allergic rhinitis, chronic rhinosinusitis, and nasal polyposis. Their effects are mediated by glucocorticoid receptor-alpha. Upon binding GC, activated GR-α enhances transcription of anti-inflammatory genes and interacts with other proteins regulating inflammation, such as nuclear factor-kappaB (NF-KB).[1] In recent years, increased understanding of intranasal corticosteroid and glucocorticoid receptor pharmacology has enabled the development of molecules designed specifically to achieve potent, localized activity with minimal risk of systemic exposure. However, an easy, simple and convenient method to evaluate the efficacy of intranasal corticosteroid has not been established yet.

Comet assay is originally developed as genotoxicity examination of industrial chemicals, agrochemicals and pharmaceuticals.[2-4] The name originates from a comet seen in the night sky. Once DNA is injured, the damaged DNA is subdivided and visible just like a tail of a comet in the electric gel.[5,6] There are some examples of applied the comet assay to evaluate the gene damage at the time of UV irradiation or γ-radiation.[2] However, the comet assay has not been applied for investigations of nasal disorders.

To clarify this point, the infiltrating cells of the patients with nasal disorders including allergic rhinitis, chronic rhinosinusitis and hyposmia were examined by comet assay. The effects of dexamethasone on DNA damage of lymphocytes obtained from normal control were also examined.

Subjects

Forty-eight patients with allergic rhinitis, 19 patients with chronic rhinitis and nine patients with hyposmia were enrolled in this study. A nasal smear was collected from each patient and the degree of DNA damage was evaluated by comet assay.[2-6]

Lymphocytes

PBL were separated from heparinized blood of collaborators which had been drawn on the previous day, and kept in 4°C until use. Lymphocytes were separated from erythrocytes and granulocytes by Lymphocytes Separation Solution (Nacalai Tesque Ltd.) (d = 1.077). Separated lymphocytes were exchanged to a RPMI-1640 culture medium (Wako) with L- glutamine and phenol red after washing twice with D-PBS (-) (for Cell Incubation, WAKO 045-29795). The cell concentration was adjusted to 2×10^6 cells/ml and used for cell culture immediately. The viability of the lymphocytes was 85%-90%.

Cell culture

One hundred μl of 2.0 x 10^6 cells/μl lymphocytes were dispensed into wells of flat-bottom 24-well plates (No. 662160, CELLSTAR Greiner bio-one). Different concentrations of DEX (Sigma company D4902 Lot # BCBD 9732V) were prepared. An equivalent quantity (100 μl) of DEX solution was put in each well of 24-well plates. Lymphocytes were maintained at 37°C in a humidified atmosphere of 5% CO_2 and 95% air. UV at 254 nm was irradiated for 20 seconds after the incubation. A UVS-14 EL series UV lamp with an Hg-law lamp was used for the UV-irradiation treatment. The amount of UV at 254 nm irradiated from 7.6 cm distance is 0.785 μW/cm² and the expected amount of UV-irradiated for 20 seconds was calculated to be 15 μJ/cm².

Comet assay

The OxiSelect™ Comet Assay Kit (Cat NO. STA-350, Cell BioLabs, Inc.) was used for the comet assay. One percent agarose solution was warmed and melted previously, and 1 ml of the solution was put on the slide glass and solidified, then 14-mm diameter holes were made for the lymphocytes solutions. Five to 10 μl of the treated lymphocytes were mixes with 90 μl of 1% agarose (Nacalai Tesque, Inc. (Cat V2111, Lot 23007901, Analytical Grade). The mixed agarose solutions were put in the wells of the slide glass. Then it was treated with cell lysis buffer (Lysis buffer (kit providing) with NaCl 14.6 g and 20 ml of 500 mM EDTA and 90 ml of distilled water) for 50 min at 4°C in the dark. It was electrophoresed after having been substituted to an alkaline buffer for 30 min. Mupid-2 plus of Advance Co., Ltd. was used for the electrophoresis under the condition of 50V, 4 min. Treated agarose was then washed three times with distilled water, substituted with 99% ethanol and dried. Vista Green DNA staining solution by diluting 1:10,000 in TE buffer (10 mM Tris, pH 7.5 and 1 mM EDTA) was used for staining DNA. The treated samples were stained for 15 min by the solution. A fluorescent microscope (Laika Microsystems Co. Ltd, DMI3000B) with fluorescent cube L5 (exitation filter BP480/40, dichroic mirror RKP505 and absorption filter BP527/30) was used for observation.

Results

Intact DNA did not make a comet-like tail (Fig. 1a), damaged DNA made a comet-like tail by comet assay (Fig. 1b). To investigate what kind of cells in the smear were stained by the comet assay, we used the double-staining technique to treat agarose. DNA was stained in green, eosinophil cationic protein in red, and CD3 in blue (Fig. 2a,b). This figure shows lymphocyte and eosinophil presence in nasal smear.

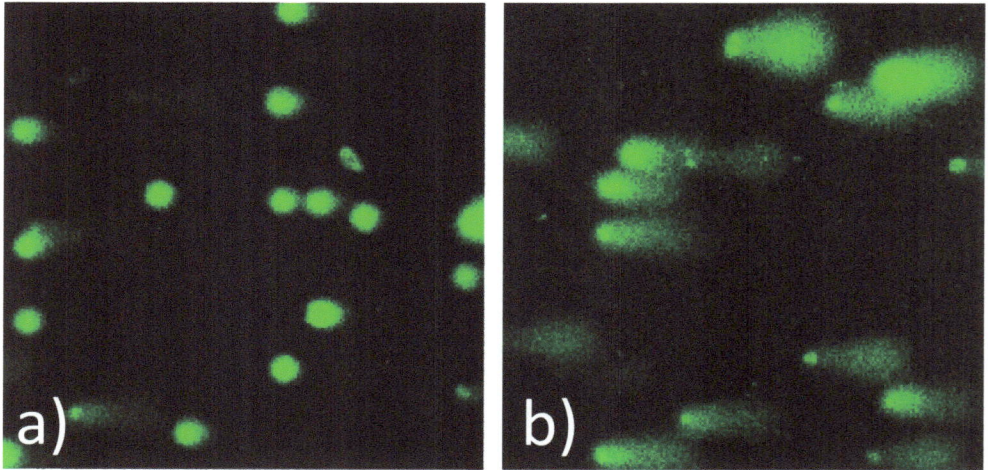

Fig. 1. Representative microscopic appearances of comet assay. Control cell (a) and DNA-damaged cell (b) in the nasal smear from patient with hyposimia and allergic rhinitis. (Comet assay, original magnification x200.)

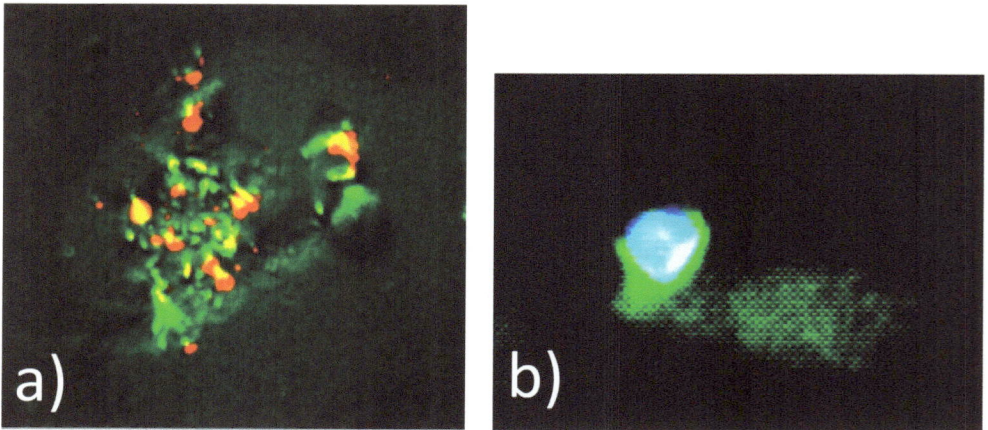

Fig. 2. MBP and Comet assay positive cell (a) and CD3 and comet assay positive cell (b) in the nasal smear obtained from patients with allergic rhinitis. (Comet assay, original magnification x200.)

The infiltrating cells of the patients with chronic sinusitis showed a higher proportion of damaged cells by comet assay than those with allergic rhinitis and hyposmia, but there was no significant difference (Fig. 3).

The infiltrating cells of the patients with nasal polyp showed a comparable proportion of damaged cells by comet assay to those with no nasal polyp (Fig. 4).

The infiltrating cells of the patients who used nasal topical steroids showed a lower proportion of damaged cells than those of the patients who used anti-histamine drugs or leukotriene antagonists, but there was no significant difference (Fig. 5).

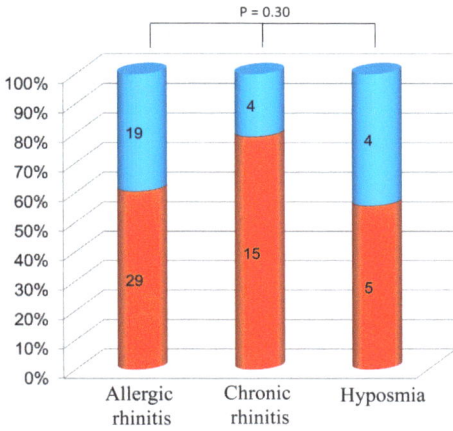

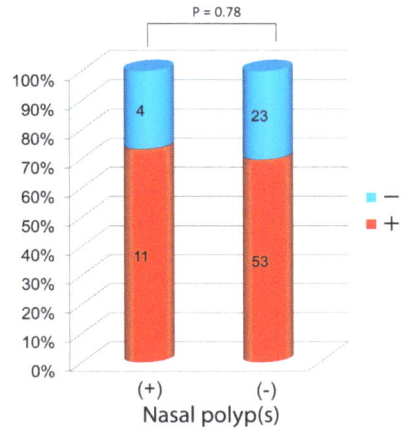

Fig. 3. Positive ratio of DNA-damaged cell and nasal disorders. The infiltrating cells of the patients with chronic sinusitis showed a higher proportion of damaged cells by comet assay than those with allergic rhinitis and hyposmia (no significant difference). Positive (red square) and negative (blue square) status in nasal smear by comet assay.

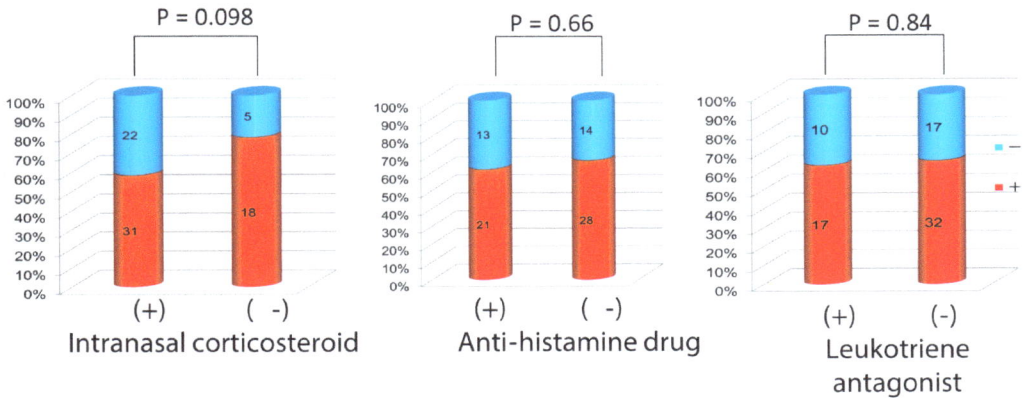

Fig. 4. Positive ratio of DNA-damaged cell in nasal smear from patients with chronic rhinosinusitis with or without nasal polyps. The infiltrating cells of the patients with chronic sinusitis showed a higher proportion of damaged cells by comet assay than those with allergic rhinitis and hyposmia (no significant difference). Positive (red square) and negative (blue square) status in nasal smear by comet assay.

Fig. 5. Positive ratio of DNA-damaged cell and treatments. The infiltrating cells of the patients who used nasal topical steroids showed a lower proportion of damaged cells than those of the patients who used antihistamine drugs or leukotriene antagonists (no significant difference). Positive (red square) and negative (blue square) status in nasal smear by comet assay.

A comet-like tail was not seen after the comet assay in samples of freshly-prepared peripheral blood lymphocytes. The comet-like tail was seen in all lymphocytes irradiated with UV-C for 20 seconds (15 μJ/cm^2) or more. We set the irradiation time at 20 seconds and investigated whether DEX was related to

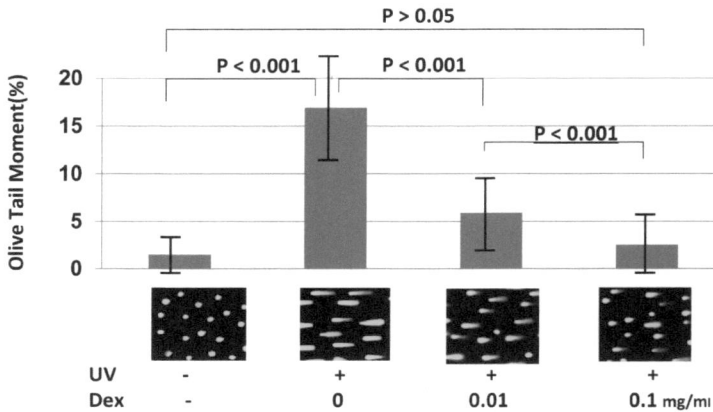

Fig. 6. The effect of dexamethasone on comet assay. PBM cultured in the presence or absence of dexamethasone. PBM were incubated in various concentrations (0.01 and 0.1 mg/ml) of dexamethasone for 12 h, whereafter DNA-damaged cells were counted by comet assay. Data are expressed as the mean ± SE (n = 13).

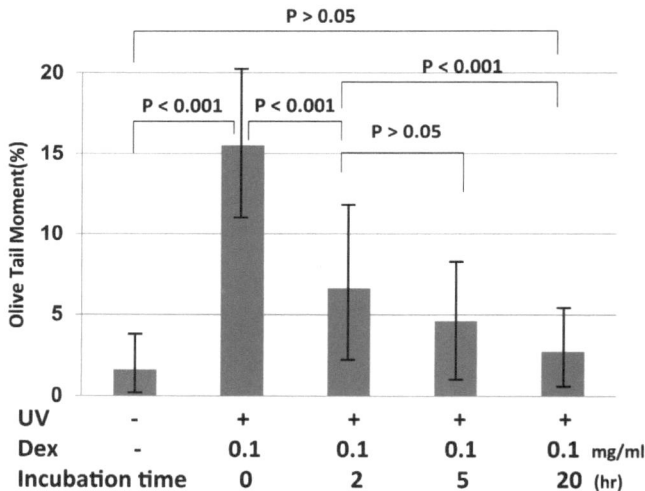

Fig. 7. Various exposure times to dexamethasone and comet assay. After BML were incubated with dexamethasone (0.1 mg/ml) for various exposure periods (two, five and 20 h), cells were washed and incubated in RPMI medium containing 10% FCS. After incubation, olive-tail moments were counted. Data are expressed as the mean ± SE (n = 12).

inhibit DNA damage on this condition. Figure 1 shows comet images obtained from incubation for 20 hours. Almost all DNAs of the lymphocytes which had not received UV irradiation were undamaged. On the other hand, the comet-like tails were seen in almost all lymphocytes incubated without DEX which had received UV irradiation. In cases of incubation with DEX, some lymphocytes showed no comet tails in any concentration and other lymphocytes showed tails in various lengths. Figure 6 shows the results of examining an effective concentration of DEX. The vertical axis is the Olive-tail moment (%). It became minimal when the concentration of DEX was 0.1 mg/ml examined between 0.01 mg/ml and 1.0 mg/ml. A significant difference was seen between 0.01 mg/ml and 0.1 mg/ml, and between 0.1 mg/ml and 1 mg/ml ($p < 0.001$). However, no significant difference was seen between 0.01 mg/ml and 1 mg/ml ($p > 0.05$). Figure 7 shows the effective time for the treatment of DEX. The lymphocytes were incubated for two hours, five hours, and 20 hours. The effect of DEX became remarkable when the incubation time was lengthened and the rate of cells showing comet-like tails decreased. The most remarkable difference was seen after incubation for 20 hours (Fig. 7).

Discussion

Comet assay provides a simple and effective method for evaluating DNA damage in cells. The samples are electrophoresed in a horizontal chamber to separate intact DNA from damaged fragments. The damaged DNA (containing cleavage and strand breaks) will migrate further than intact DNA and produce a comet-tail shape (Fig. 1).

Eosinophil cationic protein (ECP) is a marker of eosinophil, and CD3 is a marker of lymphocyte. Figure 2 shows lymphocyte and eosinophil presence in nasal smear. Chronic sinusitis and allergic rhinitis have the background of intractable, protracted chronic inflammation. So, there are macrophage, dendritic cell, plasma cell and neutrophil in nasal smear besides lymphocyte and eosinophil.

The inflammatory cells discharge various cytokines and histamine. TNF-α (tumor necrosis factor-α), as an inflammatory cytokine, induces iNOS (inducible nitric oxide synthase). INOS produces a stack of NO (nitric oxide). It is known that NO produces ONOO- and induces DNA damage by oxidative stress. DNA damaged cells were confirmed in nasal smears of patients with chronic inflammation including chronic rhinitis, allergic rhinitis and hyposmia (Fig. 3). DNA damage is induced by oxidative stress. Oxidative stress occurs in many allergic and immunologic disorders. Oxidative stress occurs not only as a result of inflammation, but also from environmental exposure to air pollution and cigarette smoke.[16] Chronic sinusitis may be an more severe inflammation than allergic rhinitis and hyposmia. However, nasal polyps hardly have any relation with DNA damage (Fig. 4).

Allergic rhinitis is treated with intranasal corticosteroid, anti-histamines and/or leukotriene antagonists frequently. Corticosteroid inhibits mast cell, eosinophil and lymphocyte infiltration into nasal mucosa. Corticosteroid inhibits production of cytokine, vascular permeability, and production of leukotriene and prostaglandin, as well. In comparison with oral corticosteroids, topical corticosteroids have fewer and milder adverse effects overall. Anti-histamine blocks the binding of histamine to its receptors. It suppresses the histamine-induced nasal discharge, sneeze and nasal congestion. Leukotriene antagonist blocks the binding of leukotriene to its receptors on endocapillary cells and eosinophils. It suppresses leukotriene-induced vasodilatory effects, vascular permeability and eosinophil chemotactic activity. Figure 5 shows that corticosteroid may reduce DNA damage of intranasal inflammatory cells (although there is no significant difference), and the pharmacological functions of anti-histamine and leukotriene antagonist have hardly any relation with the DNA damage. It has been reported that steroid protected cells from DNA damage.[4] However, the effect of steroid, anti-histamine and leukotriene antagonist protection against DNA damage remains unclear.

The present study shows DEX protects from 15 μJ/cm² of UV-C (254 nm) irradiation induced DNA damage of PBL. The damage decreased as the treatment time was lengthened. The most effective time for the treatment was found to be 20 hours and the most effective concentration was 0.1 mg/ml. The DNA damages of the lymphocytes incubated with 0.1 mg/ml DEX for 20 hours decreased with about 70% compared to those without DEX treatment.

Baumeister *et al.*[4] observed while using comet assay that DEX protects cells from hydrogen peroxide-induced DNA damage using biopsied human mini-organ culture from fresh nasal mucosa. They indicated that the oxidative DNA damages decreased with about 45% when pre-incubated with DEX for five days at 20 μM. Scoltock *et al.*[8] showed that DEX pretreated rat hepatoma cells inhibit UV-C-induced apoptosis. The cells were treated with 90 μJ/cm² of UV-C and the percentage of cells with apoptotic features by flow cytometry was determined. About 15% of rat hepatoma cells without DEX treatment had degraded DNA and about 5% of rat hepatoma cells pretreated with DEX in 24 hours before apoptosis induction. The rate of cells with damaged DNA can be decreased by treatment with DEX before apoptosis induction.

DEX may protect the DNA damage caused by any kind of stress (UV-C, hydrogen peroxide) or over the species of animal (rat hepatoma cell, human nasal mucosa cell, PBL). Oxidative stress is a causative agent in the UV activation of the p53 pathway.[9] Not only human but also marine life (the Atlantic cod (*Gadus morhua*)[10] and sea urchin (*Echinus melo*)) embryos[11] express high concentrations of the transcriptional activator p53 in response to DNA damage when exposed to UV-B radiation. It seems likely the mechanism which lies on the bottom is the same in the animal species.

Zhai *et al.*[13] suggested that in human RSa cells GRP78/BiP plays a protective role against UV-C-induced cell death, possibly via nucleotide excision repair. GRP78/BiP is a heat shock protein belonging to the HspA family. It participates in protein folding and makes the tolerance over heat form. DEX inhibited the expression of inflammatory cytokine. Yamazaki *et al.*[14] suggested that DEX reduces the expression of inflammatory cytokine by inhibiting NF-kB. DEX treatment inhibited sepsis-induced hepatic NF-kB activation by 23%.[15] Because of these results, NF-kB was also involved in the course of DEX treatment.

We used comet assay for the investigation of DNA damage of PBL. The comet assay is a good technique for examining the damage of DNA in a brief examination. Apoptosis can generate the typical comet images as soon as the cells enter the apoptosis process.[12] Recent progress of new apo/necro-Comet-assay[1] can distinguish viable, apoptotic and necrotic cells. The new technique reduces the sometimes mentioned problem of false-positive results in genotoxicity researchers. Since comet assay is an easy method of achieving results in a short time, it is useful for the elucidation of the involved mechanisms.

Conclusions

DNA damaged cells were confirmed in nasal smears of patients with chronic inflammation including chronic rhinitis, allergic rhinitis and hyposmia. DNA damage is induced by oxidative stress. Oxidative stress occurs in many allergic and immunologic disorders. Oxidative stress occurs not only as a result of in-flammation but also from environmental exposure to air pollution and cigarette smoke. Steroid has a protective effect against DNA damage dose-dependently and time-dependently. Steroid inhibits an activity of prostaglandin, leukotriene and nuclear factor-kappa B. These inhibition makes anti-inflammatory effects. The anti-DNA-damage effect of steroids seemed to play a role in this anti-inflammatory effect as well.

Acknowledgements

This work was supported by a Grant-in-Aid for Scientific Research (B), grant number 24791743, from the Japan Society for the Promotion of Science and the Ministry of Health, Labor, and Welfare of Japan. We express our sincere thanks to Mrs. Yuko Ohta, Uyo Gakuen college, for her editorial assistance.

References

1. Ishida A, Ohta N, Koike S, Aoyagi M, Yamakawa M. Overexpression of glucocorticoid receptor-beta in severe allergic rhinitis. Auris Nasus Larynx 2010;37:584-588.
2. Osipov AN, Vorobyova NYu. Comet assay study of DNA breakage and apoptosis in mice exposed to low dose-rate ionizing radiation. In: Proceedings of the 2nd Environmental physics conference, Alexandria, Egypt, 2006;197-202.
3. Matsunaga T, Hieda K, Nikaido O. Wavelength dependent formation of thimine dimmers and (6-4) photoproducts in DNA by monochromatic ultraviolet light ranging from 150 to 365 nm. Photochem Photobiol 1991;54:403-410.
4. Baumeister P, Korn, G, Berghaus A, Matthias C, Harreus U. Chemopreventive action of DEX and alpha-tocopherol in oxidative stressed cells. Cancer Detect Prev 2009;32:452-457.
5. Zibera C, Gibelli N, Butti G, et al. Proliferative effect of DEX on a human glioblastoma cell line (HU 197) is mediated by glucocorticoid receptors. Anticancer Res 1992;12:1571-1574.
6. Kawamura A, Tamaki N, Kokunai T. Effect of DEX on cell proliferation of neuroepithelial tumor cell lines. Neurol Med Chir (Tokyo) 1998;38:633-640.
7. Thoma F. Light and dark in chromatin repair: repair of UV-induced DNA lesions by photolyse and nucleotide excision repair. The EMBO Journal 1999;18:6585-6598.

8. Scoltock AB, Heimlich G, Cidlowski JA. Glucocorticoids inhibit the apoptotic actions of UV-C but not Fas ligand in hepatoma cells: direct evidence for a critical role of Bcl-xL. Cell Death Differ 2007;14:840-850.

9. Renzing J, Hansen S, Lane DP. Oxidative stress is involved in the UV activation of p53. J Cell Sci 1996;109:1105-1112.

10. Lesser MP, Farrell JH, Walker CW. Oxidative stress, DNA damage and p53 expression in the larvae of atlantic cod (Gadus morhua) exposed to ultraviolet (290-400nm) radiation. J Exp Biol 2001;204:157-164.

11. Lesser MP, Kruse V A, Barry TM. Exposure to ultraviolet radiation causes apoptosis in developing sea urchin embryos. J Exp Bio 2003;206:4097-4103.

12. Choucroun P, Gillet D, Dorange G, Sawicki B, Dewitte JD. Comet assay and early apoptosis. Mutat Res 2001;478:89-96.

13. Zhai L, Kita K, Wano C, Wu Y, Sugaya S, Suzuki N. Decreased cell survival and DNA repair capacity after UVC irradiation in association with down-regulation of GRP78/BiP in human RSa cells. Exp Cell Res 2005;305:244-252.

14. Yamazaki T, Tukiyama T, Tokiwa T. Effect of DEX on binding activity of transcription factors nuclear factor-kB and activator protein-1 in SW982 human synovial sarcoma cells. In Vitro Cel Dev Bio-Animal 2005;41:80-82.

15. Chang CK, Llanes S, Schumer W. Effect of DEX on NF-kB Activation, Tumor Necrosis Factor Formation, and Glucose Dyshomeostasis in Septic Rats. J Surg Res 1997;72:141-145.

16. Bowler RP, Crapo JD. Oxidative stress in allergic respiratory diseases. J Allergy Clin Immunol 2002;110(3):349-356.

PERSONAL EXPERIENCE IN OLFACTORY DYSFUNCTION IN PARKINSON DISEASE

Giulio Cesare Passali[1], Lucrezia Vargiu[1], Roberta Anzivino[1], Mario Rigante[1], Jacopo Galli[1], Francesco Bove[2], Anna Rita Bentivoglio[2], Alfonso Fasano[3], Eugenio De Corso[1], Monica Giuliani[1], Gaetano Paludetti[1]

[1]Department of Head and Neck Surgery, Institute of Otorhinolaryngology, Catholic University, Rome, Italy; [2]Department of Neurology, Catholic University, Rome, Italy; [3]University of Toronto, Movement Disorders Centre, Toronto Western Hospital, Toronto, Canada

Introduction

Parkinson's disease (PD) is a movement disorder characterized by bradykinesia, rigidity, rest tremor, and postural instability. However, it is recognized that PD is associated with a variety of non-motor features,[1] like gastrointestinal (GI) and smell dysfunction (which often occur years prior to the onset of motor symptoms[2] in at least 90% of cases[3,4]). Braak *et al.* described the PD neurodegeneration staging through the progressive ascending distribution of misfolded α-synuclein from the brainstem to the cortex[5] (in six steps). Braak's ascending staging model prompts the question whether the disorder might originate outside the central nervous system (CNS), caused by a yet unidentified pathogen,[6] able to pass the nasal and GI mucosal barrier, entering the anterior olfactory nucleus or the enteric neurons through a retrograde axonal transport.[7,8] This model could explain the high prevalence of non-motor symptoms, and their onset prior to motor symptoms. Our challenge in this study is to demonstrate that hypo-anosmia and GI dysfunction should have similar origins, onset and evolution across the disease stages of PD.

Address for correspondence: Dr. Giulio Cesare Passali, Department of Head and Neck Surgery, Institute of Otorhinolaryngology, Catholic University of Sacred Heart, Largo A. Gemelli 8, 00168, Rome, Italy. Tel:+390630154439. Fax: +39063051194.
E-mail: giulio.passali@rm.unicatt.it

Recent Advances in Rhinosinusitis and Nasal Polyposis, pp. 127-134
Edited by Hideyuki Kawauchi, Desiderio Passali, Ranko Mladina, Andrey Lopatin and Dmytro Zabolotnyi
2015 © Kugler Publications, Amsterdam, The Netherlands

Patients and methods

Seventy-eight outpatients were enrolled, fulfilling three inclusion criteria: diagnosis of PD according to the UK Brain Bank criteria,[9] informed consent, olfactory test. Exclusion criteria were: signs of dementia (DSM-IV criteria), score $\leq$ 26 at the Mini-Mental-State-Examination, head trauma, neurological, nasal or systemic disorders potentially affecting olfactory function.

Motor condition was assessed by Hoehn and Yahr staging[10] and by section III of the Unified PD Rating Scale, UPDRS-III, (in off and on conditions). Patients were studied through the Sniffin' Sticks® olfactory test (Burghart instruments, Germany), performing olfactory threshold, detection and identification test.[11] The test was preceded by rhinomanometry,[12] sensitized with nasal decongestion. The overall score of the three tests, TDI score (threshold, Discrimination, Identification) was calculated (range from 0 to 48). TDI values < 15 identify anosmic subjects,[13] while values < 5 are not reliable.

Enrolled patients were questioned about the occurrence of non-motor symptoms. The interview was performed in a structured fashion using an in-house standardized worksheet developed by another group.[14] It consisted of 24 specific questions to assess the presence of non-motor symptoms, concerning olfaction, vision, psychiatric and cognitive status, sleep, autonomic dysfunction, GI symptoms.

For any affirmative answer, participants were asked to report the time of symptom's onset. Positive familiar history for PD, age at onset, disease duration, motor phenotype at PD onset, therapy, smoking habit and number of weekly evacuation were also assessed.

Results

Seventy-eight PD patients were enrolled (50 males and 28 females; age: 69.7 $\pm$ 9.2 years; disease duration: 11.1 $\pm$ 5.4 years, Hoehn and Yahr stage: 2.1 $\pm$ 0.6). Thirty-one patients (39.4%) were smokers, without inter-groups differences ($p = 0.4$).

Threshold, discrimination, identification scores were: 3.2 $\pm$ 2.7, 8.3 $\pm$ 3.0 and 8.2 $\pm$ 2.5, respectively; TDI mean score was 19.7 $\pm$ 7.5. Olfactory dysfunction was objectively detected in 91.0% of patients, a percentage higher than subjective hyposmia declared (55.1%; $p < 0.0001$). Seven patients (9.0%) were normosmic, 49 (62.8%) hyposmic, 22 (28.2%) anosmic. These three subgroups differed in gender distribution ($p = 0.005$), age at disease onset ($p = 0.04$) and, as statistical trend, disease duration ($p = 0.057$)(Table 1).

Post-hoc analysis showed that the percentage of males was lower in anosmic than hyposmic ($p = 0.003$) and normosmic group ($p = 0.03$); age at disease onset was lower in normosmic than hyposmic ($p = 0.04$) and anosmic ($p = 0.02$) group.

The occurrence of non-motor symptoms in normosmic, hyposmic and anosmic patients did not differ across groups, with the exception of subjective hyposmia

Table 1. Demographic and clinical data of patients. Bolt-typed values are significantly different across groups.

	Total	*Anosmic*	*Hyposmic*	*Normosmic*
Number	78	22	49	7
Male/female (ratio)	**50/28**	**8/14**[a]	**36/13**	**6/1**
Age	65.5 ± 9.1	68.1 ± 7.8	64.2 ± 9.8	66.1 ± 7.4
Age at onset	**58.6 ± 10.1**	**62.8 ± 7.7**	**57.4 ± 10.4**	**53.4 ± 10.7**[b]
Smokers	31 (39.7%)	6 (27.3%)	22 (44.9%)	3 (42.9%)
Familiar history of PD	9 (11.5%)	1 (4.5%)	8 (16.3%)	0 (0%)
Hoehn & Yahr stage	2.1 ± 0.6	2.0 ± 0.6	2.1 ± 0.6	2.3 ± 0.3
UPDRS-III total score med ON	16.5 ± 6.3	15.4 ± 6.6	17.1 ± 6.5	16.0 ± 3.2
UPDRS-III total score med OFF	24.7 ± 8.0	22.4 ± 7.4	25.3 ± 8.2	27.6 ± 7.2
Threshold	**3.2 ± 2.7**	**1.0 ± 1.1**[c]	**3.7 ± 2.5**[d]	**7.0 ± 2.1**
Identification	8.3 ± 3.0	5.4 ± 2.1[e]	9.0 ± 2.3[f]	12.4 ± 1.3
Discrimination	8.2 ± 3.5	4.9 ± 1.7[g]	9.0 ± 2.9[h]	13.3 ± 2.2
TDI score	19.7 ± 7.5	11.1 ± 3.0[i]	21.7 ± 4.9[j]	32.7 ± 1.9

[a]: different than hyposmic (p=0.003) and normosmic group (p = 0.03); [b]: different than hyposmic (p = 0.04), and anosmic (p = 0.02) group; [c]: different than hyposmic (p < 0.001) and normosmic group (p < 0.001); [d]: different than normosmic group (p = 0.003); [e]: different than hyposmic (p < 0.001) and normosmic group (p < 0.001); [f]: different than normosmic group (p < 0.001); [g]: different than hyposmic (p < 0.001) and normosmic group (p < 0.001); [h]: different than normosmic group (p = 0.001); [i]: different than hyposmic (p < 0.001) and normosmic group (p < 0.001); [j]: different than normosmic group (p < 0.001).

(p = 0.007), constipation (0.01), number of bowel movements/week (p = 0.03), bloating (p = 0.04) and dyspepsia (p = 0.05). On post-hoc analysis, constipation prevalence in patients with anosmia and hyposmia was higher than in normosmic ones (72.7% and 69.4% vs. 14.3%; p = 0.006 and p = 0.005, respectively). The number of bowel moments/week was higher in normosmic patients (6.7 ± 0.8) than anosmic (5.0 ± 1.8, p = 0.04) and hyposmic patients (4.9 ± 3.0, p = 0.01). Bloating was higher in anosmic and hyposmic than in normosmic patients (54.5% and 40.8% vs. 0%; p = 0.03 and p = 0.01, respectively) and dyspepsia was higher in anosmic than hyposmic patients (54.5% vs. 28.5%, p = 0.05).

As for age at onset of the different non-motor symptoms, no significant differences arose (Table 2).

TDI did not correlate with any continuous demographical and clinical data. Threshold and discrimination did not show correlations, identification correlates with age (R = -0.23, p = 0.04) and age at disease onset (R = -0.27, p = 0.02).

Discussion

Our study confirms the high frequency of olfactory and GI dysfunctions in PD patients.

Table 2. Age at onset of non-motor symptoms.

	N =	Total	Anosmic	Hyposmic	Normosmic
Disturbance of colour vision	4	63.7 ± 15.3	75.0	60.0 ± 16.4	
Crying during sleep	13	65.1 ± 10.0	70.0 ± 6.0	63.6 ± 10.8	
Nightmares	24	63.5 ± 9.3	65.0 ± 10.8	63.4 ± 9.2	55.0
Vivid dreams	36	62.7 ± 10.7	64.2 ± 12.1	62.5 ± 10.6	55.0
Limb movements during sleep	33	63.4 ± 11.7	68.7 ± 7.9	62.1 ± 12.4	57.0
Problems with staying asleep	47	63.5 ± 10.5	68.5 ± 7.8	61.3 ± 11.3	61.7 ± 4.9
Falling asleep	40	63.2 ± 11.6	69.0 ± 8.4	62.4 ± 11.4	53.7 ± 14.2
Subjective hyposmia	41	62.0 ± 11.0	65.3 ± 10.4	59.5 ± 11.3	62.0
Constipation	51	63.3 ± 11.1	63.6 ± 12.7	63.3 ± 10.7	60.0
Diarrhea	1	69.0	69.0		
Alternate bowel	3	58.3 ± 21.2	73.0	51.0 ± 24.0	
Bloating	32	61.6 ± 13.6	64.6 ± 11.0	59.8 ± 15.0	
Abdominal pain	22	61.8 ± 10.6	63.2 ± 14.6	61.4 ± 9.7	
Dyspepsia	27	60.9 ± 9.5	63.3 ± 12.7	59.0 ± 5.9	58.0
Increased sweating	18	60.9 ± 9.4	61.3 ± 3.4	60.7 ± 11.5	
Seborrhea	6	62.3 ± 8.1	62.5 ± 6.4	62.2 ± 9.9	
Orthostatic dizziness	25	65.0 ± 7.0	67.6 ± 3.1	63.2 ± 8.0	71.0
Anxiety	41	61.7 ± 13.3	63.9 ± 12.1	60.2 ± 14.9	63.0 ± 5.8
Moodiness	19	62.6 ± 9.0	68.7 ± 9.0	60.3 ± 9.4	63.3 ± 2.3
Depression	38	63.7 ± 9.4	68.2 ± 9.2	61.4 ± 9.2	63.7 ± 6.7
Apathy	27	61.9 ± 13.3	69.2 ± 8.0	57.9 ± 15.1	63.7 ± 6.7
Problem to recall name	42	62.3 ± 14.0	67.7 ± 7.8	61.1 ± 12.6	50.5 ± 29.8
Forgetfulness and finding of words	45	62.9 ± 12.2	67.9 ± 6.2	62.6 ± 9.6	50.5 ± 29.8
Bradyphrenia	33	61.2 ± 13.0	69.0 ± 7.2	59.0 ± 14.3	59.7 ± 5.5

What we found is the direct link between them, as GI dysfunctions are more represented in hyposmic/anosmic patients.

This finding supports the Braak's PD staging model[15] and the hypothesis of the existence of environmental agents able to directly damage the olfactory and GI systems together.

We found an olfaction impairment in the 91.0% of patients.[16] Interestingly, the 35.9% of patients were unaware of the smell disorder, thus suggesting the importance of a routine clinical assessment to detect it.[11] Constipation, after hyposmia, was the most frequent non-motor symptom (65.4% of patients).[17]

There might be a direct involvement of the enteric nervous system, demonstrated by the identification of Lewy bodies and loss of dopaminergic neurons[18,19] in the peripheral nervous system and in the dorsal motor nucleus of the vagus nerve.[20-21] Non-myelinated or sparsely myelinated neurons with disproportionately long and thin axons (as olfactory receptor neurons, mitral and tufted cells[22]) are susceptible to the aggregations and misfoldings of α-synuclein.[23] These cells are prone to oxidative stress and neurodegeneration. These observations led Braak and colleagues to hypothesize that PD starts outside the CNS, caused by environmental agents (prions, viruses, metals, solvents, pesticides[24-26]). Genetic substrates may interact with environmental factors to induce most forms of sporadic PD.[27] PD could be caused by pathogens penetrating the brain via the olfactory and/or vagal fibers from the nervous enteric plexa, resulting in GI and smell dysfunctions secondary to damage to the olfactory and motor brain regions.[28-30] In all patients, olfaction impairment and GI involvement are correlated: for instance, more than 70% of hypo/anosmic patients presented constipation, in contrast with the 14.3% observed in the normosmic ones, a prevalence similar to the general adult healthy population.[31] Another novel aspect is the characterization of a subgroup of normosmic patients, with early diagnosis of PD, in these patients the contribution of genetic abnormalities might be greater, and the role of external toxic agents marginal, so the disease probably starts directly inside the CNS;[32,33] accordingly a normal olfactory threshold and no GI symptom were detected.

We also found an inverse correlation between TDI and age at disease onset in the whole sample of patients.

Our study has some limitations. The group of normosmic patients is small (seven) (even if statistically significant correlations were found). None of these patients underwent genetic analysis, but the onset in younger age of PD may be an argument in favor of the genetic contribution. The possibility of false-negative normosmic patients is very unlikely since we used a 'sensitized' olfactory test (rhinomanometry and a nasal decongestion previously performed).[34,35] Moreover, gastrointestinal discomfort and constipation are very common chronic symptoms in general population and above all in women. Anyway to establish the exact prevalence of constipation (as well as gastrointestinal discomfort or Inflammatory Bowel Diseases, IBD) is very difficult, firstly for the overlapping symptoms of these disorders, secondly, the series conducted are based on self-reported symptoms and subjective questionnaires, and some risk factors for constipation[36] are not considered. In any case, the rate seems to be similar all over the different countries 2-28%,[37] and in Europe it should correspond to the 17%;[36,38] a series conducted in Greece (2014)[39] showed the higher prevalence of the problem in women, compared to men (21% vs. 11%), and should be correlated to alimentary habits, stress, age, etc. In the data obtained from the series of Suares,[40] the prevalence of constipation is 14% and women and people suffering of IBD, seem to be more prone to develop it, but the countries analyzed do not include Europe. It is easy to understand how difficult it is to define the prevalence of constipation, and it would be useful to analyze it with the most coherent cohort of patients possible to avoid the overlap with other disorders such as IBD.

Conclusions

In our series we found a direct link between olfactory and gastrointestinal dysfunction, thus supporting the environmental mechanism in the pathophysiology of PD[15]. This might help in establishing a screening for the early diagnosis in patients prone to develop PD, so that they could be enrolled in trials for studying new medicines to prevent it. In addition, we have characterized a very specific subgroup of patients with earlier age at onset of PD and lack of olfactory and GI problems, probably genetically predisposed.

Further series would be helpful for identifying genes responsible for PD and, above all, objective assessment of olfactory and gastrointestinal dysfunction, are needed to upgrade our knowledge of PD etiopathogenesis, to try to prevent and cure it. In order to achieve this, a very large sample of patients is needed, that would also allow the detection of a sizable number of normosmic patients.

References

1. Halliday GM, Barker RA, Rowe DB. Non-dopamine lesions in Parkinson's disease. New York: Oxford University Press, 2011.
2. Ross GW, Petrovitch H, Abbott RD, et al. Association of olfactory dysfunction with risk for future Parkinson's disease. Ann Neurol 2008;63:167-173.
3. Doty RL, Deems DA, Stellar S. Olfactory dysfunction in parkinsonism: a general deficit unrelated to neurologic signs, disease stage, or disease duration. Neurology 1988;38:1237-1244.
4. Alves G, Forsaa EB, Pedersen KF, Dreetz Gjerstad M, Larsen JP. Epidemiology of Parkinson's disease. J Neurol 2008;255 Suppl 5:18-32.
5. Braak H, Del Tredici K, Bratzke H, Hamm-Clement J, Sandmann-Keil D, Rub U. Staging of the intracerebral inclusion body pathology associated with idiopathic Parkinson's disease (preclinical and clinical stages). J Neurol 2002;249 Suppl 3:III/1-5.
6. Braak H, Del Tredici K, Rub U, de Vos RA, Jansen Steur EN, Braak E. Staging of brain pathology related to sporadic Parkinson's disease. Neurobiol of Aging 2003;24:197-211.
7. Braak H, Rub U, Gai WP, Del Tredici K. Idiopathic Parkinson's disease: possible routes by which vulnerable neuronal types may be subject to neuroinvasion by an unknown pathogen. J Neural Transm 2003;110:517-536.
8. Phillips RJ, Walter GC, Wilder SL, Baronowsky EA, Powley TL. Alpha-synuclein-immunopositive myenteric neurons and vagal preganglionic terminals: autonomic pathway implicated in Parkinson's disease? Neuroscience 2008;153:733-750.
9. Gelb DJ, Oliver E, Gilman S. Diagnostic criteria for Parkinson disease. Arch Neurol 199;56:33-39.
10. Martinez-Martin P, Gil-Nagel A, Gracia LM, Gomez JB, Martinez-Sarries J, Bermejo F. Unified Parkinson's Disease Rating Scale characteristics and structure. The Cooperative Multicentric Group. Movement Disord 1994;9:76-83.
11. Hummel T, Sekinger B, Wolf SR, Pauli E, Kobal G. 'Sniffin' sticks': olfactory performance assessed by the combined testing of odor identification, odor discrimination and olfactory threshold. Chem Senses 1997;22:39-52.
12. Ogura JH, Stokstead P. Rhinomanometry in some rhinologic diseases. Laryngoscope 1958;68:2001-2014.
13. Hummel T, Kobal G, Gudziol H, Mackay-Sim A. Normative data for the "Sniffin' Sticks" including tests of odor identification, odor discrimination, and olfactory thresholds: an upgrade based on a group of more than 3,000 subjects. Eur Arch Oto-Rhino-Laryngol 2007;264:237-243.
14. Gaenslen A, Swid I, Liepelt-Scarfone I, Godau J, Berg D. The patients' perception of prodromal symptoms before the initial diagnosis of Parkinson's disease. Movement Disord 2011;26:653-658.

15. Braak H, Ghebremedhin E, Rub U, Bratzke H, Del Tredici K. Stages in the development of Parkinson's disease-related pathology. Cell Tissue Res 2004;318:121-134.
16. Doty RL. Olfaction in Parkinson's disease and related disorders. Neurobiol Dis 2012;46:527-552.
17. Pfeiffer RF. Gastrointestinal dysfunction in Parkinson's disease. Lancet Neurol 2003;2:107-116.
18. Kupsky WJ, Grimes MM, Sweeting J, Bertsch R, Cote LJ. Parkinson's disease and mega-colon: concentric hyaline inclusions (Lewy bodies) in enteric ganglion cells. Neurology 1987;37:1253-1255.
19. Singaram C, Ashraf W, Gaumnitz EA, et al. Dopaminergic defect of enteric nervous system in Parkinson's disease patients with chronic constipation. Lancet 1995;346:861-864.
20. Gai WP, Blessing WW, Blumbergs PC. Ubiquitin-positive degenerating neurites in the brainstem in Parkinson's disease. Brain 1995;118 (Pt 6):1447-1459.
21. Halliday GM, Blumbergs PC, Cotton RG, Blessing WW, Geffen LB. Loss of brainstem sero-tonin- and substance P-containing neurons in Parkinson's disease. Brain Res 1990;510:104-107.
22. Hubbard PS, Esiri MM, Reading M, McShane R, Nagy Z. Alpha-synuclein pathology in the olfactory pathways of dementia patients. J Anatomy 2007;211:117-124.
23. Braak H, Del Tredici K. Neuroanatomy and pathology of sporadic Parkinson's disease. Adv Anat Embryol Cell Biol 2009;201:1-119.
24. McBride PA, Schulz-Schaeffer WJ, Donaldson M, et al. Early spread of scrapie from the gastrointestinal tract to the central nervous system involves autonomic fibers of the splanchnic and vagus nerves. J Virol 2001;75:9320-9327.
25. Tanner CM, Ross GW, Jewell SA, et al. Occupation and risk of parkinsonism: a multicenter case-control study. Arch Neurol 2009;66:1106-1113.
26. Elbaz A, Clavel J, Rathouz PJ, et al. Professional exposure to pesticides and Parkinson disease. Ann Neurol 2009;66:494-504.
27. Lin CH, Wu RM, Tai CH, Chen ML, Hu FC. Lrrk2 S1647T and BDNF V66M interact with environmental factors to increase risk of Parkinson's disease. Parkinsonism Relat D 2011;17:84-88.
28. Hawkes CH, Del Tredici K, Braak H. Parkinson's disease: a dual-hit hypothesis. Neuropathol Appl Neurobiol 2007;33:599-614.
29. Braak H, de Vos RA, Bohl J, Del Tredici K. Gastric alpha-synuclein immunoreactive inclu-sions in Meissner's and Auerbach's plexuses in cases staged for Parkinson's disease-related brain pathology. Neurosci Lett 2006;396:67-72.
30. Doty RL. The olfactory vector hypothesis of neurodegenerative disease: is it viable? Ann Neurol 2008;63:7-15.
31. Stewart WF, Liberman JN, Sandler RS, et al. Epidemiology of constipation (EPOC) study in the United States: relation of clinical subtypes to sociodemographic features. Amer J Gastroenterol 1999;94:3530-3540.
32. Alcalay RN, Siderowf A, Ottman R, et al. Olfaction in Parkin heterozygotes and compound heterozygotes: the CORE-PD study. Neurology 2011;76:319-326.
33. Ferraris A, Ialongo T, Passali GC, et al. Olfactory dysfunction in Parkinsonism caused by PINK1 mutations. Movement Disord 2009;24:2350-2357.
34. Passali D, Mezzedimi C, Passali GC, Nuti D, Bellussi L. The role of rhinomanometry, acoustic rhinometry, and mucociliary transport time in the assessment of nasal patency. Ear Nose Throat J 2000;79:397-400.
35. Passàli D, Lauriello M, Bellussi L. Importance of nasal secretion pH for the olfactory func-tion. In: Passàli D (Ed.), Rhinology up-to-date. Roma: Industria Grafica Romana 1994, pp. 268-271.
36. Peppas G, et al. Epidemiology of constipation in Europe and Oceania: a systematic review. BMC Gastroenterol 2008;8:5. doi: 10.1186/1471-230X-8-5.

37. Brandt LJ, Prather CM, Quigley EMM, Schiller LR, Schoenfeld P, Talley NJ. Systematic review on the management of chronic constipation in North America. Am J Gastroenterol 2005;100:S5-22.
38. Emmanuel A, et al. Factors affecting satisfaction with treatment in European women with chronic constipation: an internet survey. United European Gastroenterol J; 2013;1(5):375-384.
39. Papatheodoridis GV, et al. A Greek survey of community prevalence and characteristics of constipation. Eur J Gastroenterol Hepatol 2010;22(3):354-360.
40. Suares NC, Ford AC. Prevalence of, and risk factors for, chronic idiopathic constipation in the community: systematic review and meta-analysis. Am J Gastroenterol 2011;106(9):1582-1591;1581;1592.

MANAGEMENT OF SINONASAL INVERTED PAPILLOMA

Yuji Nakamaru, Dai Takagi and Satoshi Fukuda

Department of Otolaryngology, Head and Neck Surgery, Hokkaido University Graduate School of Medicine

Introduction

Sinonasal inverted papillomas (IPs) are rare tumors in the nasal and paranasal sinus area.[1] IPs are basically benign, but they can have aggressive features and a high rate of recurrence. As they also have a malignant transformation, thorough removal of these tumors and their attachment sites is required.[2] Because the recurrence rate of endonasal surgery was very high, two decade ago lateral rhinotomy was the Gold Standard for this tumor surgery.[1] Because of the recent development of instruments and surgical methods, endoscopic nasal surgery (ESS) has become the first choice for IP surgery. Still, there remain some cases in which we should use an external approach to resect IP, depending on the attachment site.

In this paper, we review the recent optimal management for IP, focusing on the tumor attachment sites.

Attachment-oriented surgery

There are several reasons for the high potential of recurrence of IPs. The main reason is the anatomical complexity of the nose and paranasal structures. IPs tend to invade the bone at the site of the tumor attachment which makes it hard to resect completely.

To manage the remodeling of the bone around the tumor attachment site, attachment-oriented surgery was accepted among many top nasal surgeons. The concept of this surgery is as follows. The tumor, originating from the mucosa,

Address for correspondence: Dr. Yuji Nakamaru, Department of Otolaryngology–Head and Neck Surgery, Hokkaido University Graduate bSchool of Medicine, West 7, North 15, Sapporo 060-8638, Japan. E-mail: nmaru@med.hokudai.ac.jp

Recent Advances in Rhinosinusitis and Nasal Polyposis, pp. 135-137
Edited by Hideyuki Kawauchi, Desiderio Passali, Ranko Mladina, Andrey Lopatin
and Dmytro Zabolotnyi
2015 © Kugler Publications, Amsterdam, The Netherlands

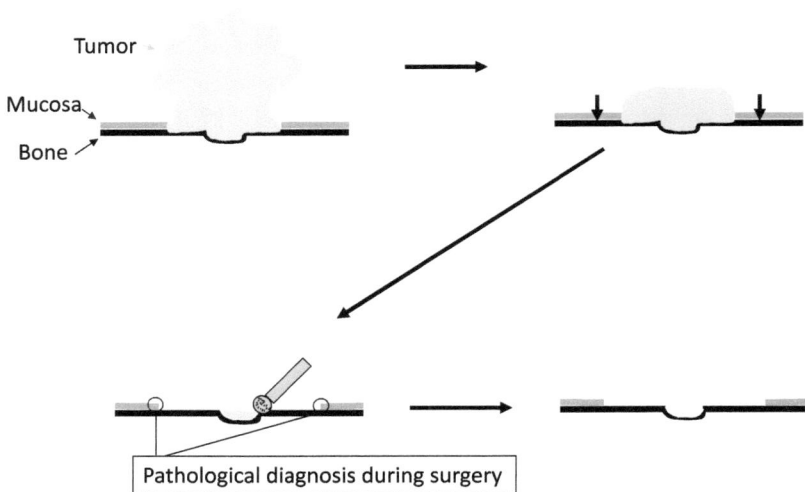

Fig. 1. Schematics of the attachment-oriented surgery. The stages are: 1) Tumor de-bulking; 2) Precise identification of the tumor's mucosal attachment; 3) Tumor dissection; 4) Excision of the tumor and its surrounding normal mucosa; 5) Resection or drilling of the bone around the attachment site with a diamond burr.

de-bulked until the tumor attachment site can be identified. Then the tumor is resected with a safety margin, making sure by pathological diagnosis during surgery it is resected completely. The remaining tumor is drilled away with a diamond burr[2] (Fig. 1).

In attachment-oriented surgery, an appropriate approach to obtain good surgical fields is needed. Although the approach may vary depending on surgical skill and available equipment, ESS may be chosen for a tumor attached at the nasal cavity, medial, upper and wall of the maxillary sinus, ethmoid, and sphenoid sinus. A tumor attached to the inferior and lateral wall of the maxillary sinus can be managed with endoscopic medial maxillectomy (EMM). A tumor attached to the frontal sinus and supraorbital cell requires an external approach. Surgical approach should be adapted to the tumor attachment site.[3] To identify the tumor attachment site is mandatory for a complete resection.

Preoperative imagings

There have been some attempts to identify the tumor attachment site. Most of these attempts were examined by C.T. Bhalla who reported that otitis signs such as thickening and resorption of the bone existed in 63-88% of IP patients.[4] These signs were exited 83-100% especially at the tumor attachment site. On the other hand, these signs also appeared at the site without tumor attachment.

Using MRI, Iimura *et al.* reported that the center of the radial structure and the opposite side of the empty space represent the tumor origin. They reported 85.7% correlation with the surgical results.[5] But there is no study reporting about sensitivity and specificity of these methods.

We have reported about the usefulness of MRI and CT as preoperative imaging for inverted papilloma surgery.[6] Ten consecutive pathologically proven IP patients underwent three Tesla (3T) MRI, 1.5 Tesla (1.5T) MRI, and CT scans preoperatively. All images were retrospectively reviewed by two radiologists. The actual tumor attachment sites were confirmed during surgery by pathological examination of the specimens.

Compared to the 3T MRI and 1.5T MRI, 3T MRI was better in all parameters than 1.5T MRI, although not significantly. MRI showed good specificity but poor sensitivity. CT showed excellent sensitivity; however, the specificity was significantly lower. CT plus MRI showed both excellent sensitivity and specificity. We concluded, therefore, that the best method to find the attachment site before surgery is to (1) search for otitis signs such as newly-generated, thickened and destructed bone using CT; (2) confirm the area around otitis sign using MRI. If the MRI shows that there is a tumor around the otitis sign, the area around otitis sign is the real tumor attachment site. If there is no tumor around the sign, it may be just a case of chronic inflammation.

Conclusion

IP is the tumor that easily recurs after surgery, which can be approached endonasally. However, this is a difficult area to manage endonasally. It is important to survey the tumor attachment site before IP surgery using CT and MRI. Precise assessment of the attachment site may be the key point to manage these tumors without recurrence.

References

1. Lawson W, Kaufman, Biller HF. Treatment outcomes in the management of inverted papilloma: an analysis of 160 cases. Laryngoscope 2003;113:1548-1556.
2. Landsberg R, Cavel O, Segev Y, Khafif A, Fliss DM. Attachment-oriented endoscopic surgical strategy for sinonasal inverted papilloma. Am J Rhinol 2008;22:629-364.
3. Oikawa K, Furuta Y, Nakamaru, Oridate N, Fukuda S. Preoperative staging and surgical approaches for sinonasal inverted papilloma. Ann Otol Rhinol Laryngol 2007;116:674-680.
4. Bhalla RK, Wright ED. Predicting the site of attachment of sinonasal inverted papilloma. Rhinology 2009;47:345-348.
5. Iimura J, Otori N, Ojiri H, Moriyama H. Preoperative magnetic resonance imaging for localization of the origin of maxillary sinus inverted papillomas. Auris Nasus Larynx 2009;36(4):416-421.
6. Nakamaru Y, Fujima N, Takagi D, A Tsukahara, Yoshida D, Fukuda S. Prediction of the Attachment Site of Sinonasal Inverted Papillomas by Preoperative Imaging Ann Otol Rhinol Laryngol 2014;123:468-474.

MACROLIDES IN CHRONIC RHINOSINUSITIS – FUTURE ASPECTS

Shoji Matsune

Nippon Medical School Musashikosugi Hospital, Department of Otolaryngology, Kawasaki City, Japan

Introduction

Macrolides belong to the family of 14- or 15-membered lactone ring antibiotics, originally found in a Philippine soil sample. These antibiotics achieve a high intracellular concentration and have a spectrum of activity against gram-positive cocci, but also intracellular pathogens such as Chlamydia and Mycoplasma.[1]

In 1984, Kudoh *et al.* reported a remarkable improvement of symptoms in 14-membered lactone ring macrolide, erythromycin (EM)-treated patients suffering from diffuse panbronchiolitis (DPB). DPB, which mainly occurs in East-Asian people, is characterized by chronic airway infection with diffuse bilateral micronodular pulmonary lesions. The advent of macrolides have a strikingly changed DPB prognosis. The bactericidal activity of macrolides is not a significant factor for their clinical efficacy in DPB; (1) irrespective of bacterial clearance, clinical improvement is observed in patients treated with EM; (2) even in cases with bacterial superinfection with *Pseudomonas aeruginosa* resistant to macrolides, treatment has proved effective; (3) the recommended dosage of macrolides produces peak levels in tissue that are below the minimum inhibitory concentrations (MIC) for major pathogenic bacteria that colonize the airway.[2,3]

Since long-term, even low-dose, macrolide therapy (macrolide therapy) turned out to be quite effective in improving survival rates in DPB cases, the mechanism of this efficacy independent of bactericidal activity of macrolides has been the research target in Japan in the field of upper and lower respiratory inflammation. Macrolide therapy was quite successfully studied in chronic rhinosinusitis as a complication of COPD.[4] In the 1990s, the effect of macrolide therapy on CRS was studied in many hospitals all over Japan, and its efficacy was confirmed

Address for correspondence: Shoji Matsune MD, PhD, Nippon Medical School, Musashikosugi Hospital, Department of Otolaryngology, Kawasaki City, Japan. E-mail: sm1988@nms.ac.jp

Recent Advances in Rhinosinusitis and Nasal Polyposis, pp. 139-145
Edited by Hideyuki Kawauchi, Desiderio Passali, Ranko Mladina, Andrey Lopatin and Dmytro Zabolotnyi
2015 © Kugler Publications, Amsterdam, The Netherlands

in many clinical trials. New 14-membered lactone ring macrolides such as clarithromycin (CAM) and roxithromycin (RXM) were produced as derivatives of EM in this decade. Major advantages of these new macrolides are as follows; (1) more acid stable and rapid absorption from gastrointestinal tract than EM; (2) less gastrointestinal side effects than EM.

Treatment dosage, period and indication

According to the guideline for macrolide treatment of chronic paranasal sinusitis (draft) in 1998, low dose means half of the usual dose as follows; 600 mg/day of EM, 200 mg/day of CAM and 150 mg /day of RXM. Long-term usually means medication for three months, and extended period for less than six months is available in effective cases. Endoscopic sinus surgery may be chosen in adult CRS cases resistant to macrolide therapy.

This medication policy is applicable in adult CRS cases. Although macrolide therapy is thought to be effective in children, many sinusitis cases in children are more affected by acute bacterial infection complicated with allergic rhinitis than in adult CRS cases. Administration of penicillin and/or antihistamine often takes priority over macrolide therapy. Macrolide therapy is thought to be a contraindication in IgE-dependent inflammation pathophysiologically.[5]

Otitis media with effusion (OME) is an additional indication, especially in cases complicated with CRS and/or epipharyngitis.[6]

Therapeutic effects of macrolides on symptoms and local findings in CRS

Many publications, in Japanese literature especially in the 1990s, attest to the benefit of macrolide therapy for the treatment of nasal manifestation. Figures 1 and 2 show the average improvement rate of symptomatic complaints (Fig. 1) and endonasal findings (Fig. 2) based on the data reported in Japanese literature published in 1995-97. While inflamed secretory components are obviously improved commonly in symptoms and endonasal status, olfaction is likely less recovered by macrolide therapy.[7]

In the meta-analysis of English-language studies, convincing evidence of clinically significant improvements have not been reported enough yet in comparison with placebos.[8] In the latest review article about macrolide therapy for CRS based on meta-analysis in the United States, it is pointed out that there is no clinically significant improvement in patient-oriented quality of life measures with long-term macrolide therapy for CRS; simultaneously, however, there may be an effect among the subgroup of patients with low serum IgE. Further studies about this scientific theme should be designed and adequately powered for a priori subgroup analysis based on IgE and other inflammatory marker profiles.

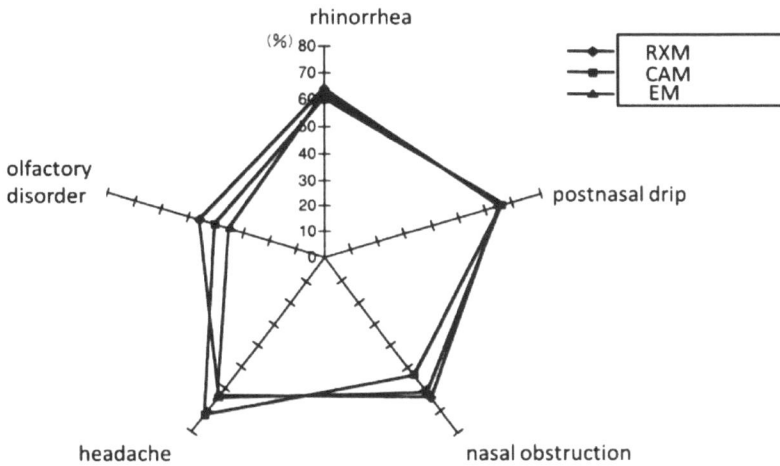

Fig. 1. Average improvement rate of symptomatic complaints published in Japanese literature in 1995~97.

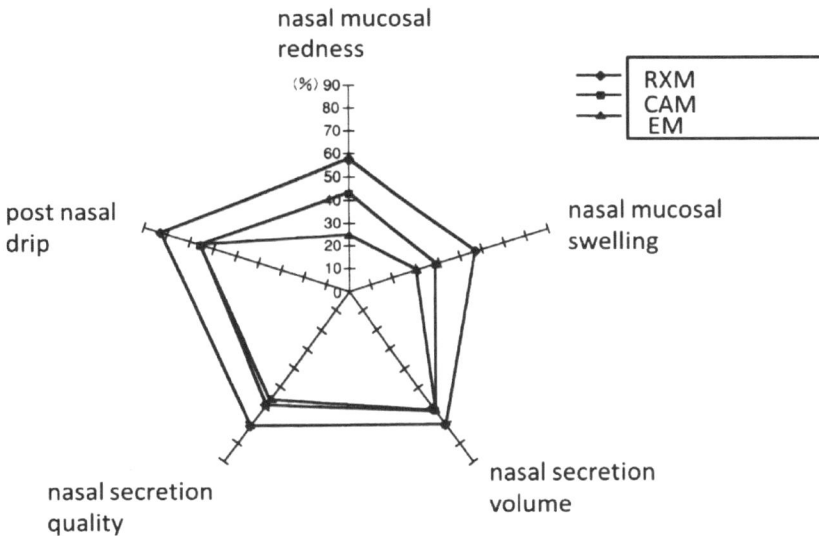

Fig. 2. Average improvement rate of nasal findings published in Japanese literature in 1995~97.

Macrolide therapy in the European Position Paper on Rhinosinusitis and Nasal Polyps 2012 (EPOS 2012)[9]

A number of open studies using macrolides have shown a response rate of 60-80%. Since in a study lacking a placebo group the risk of over-estimating efficacy of the intervention is high, placebo-controlled studies are necessary to show the efficacy of macrolide therapy. However, to date, prospective randomized placebo-controlled trials (RCT) are quite rare in macrolide therapy. Wallwork et al.[10] showed in RCT clinical effects of macrolide therapy with significant improvement in SNOT-20 score, nasal endoscopy, saccharine transit time and IL-8 levels in lavage fluid in CRS without nasal polyps after RXM 12-week medication.

Macrolide therapy should be reserved for patients where nasal corticosteroids and nasal saline irrigation have failed to reduce symptoms to an acceptable level. The population with high serum IgE are less likely to respond to macrolide therapy.

In CRS with nasal polyps, in an uncontrolled study with CAM 400mg/day for at least three months, polyps were reduced in size and IL-8 levels decreased. IL-8 levels in the group with reduced polyps were initially significantly higher before macrolide therapy than those in the group whose polyps showed no change.[11]

Anti-inflammatory mechanism of macrolide

Mechanisms of the efficacy of macrolide therapy have been regarded not as anti-microbiological, but as anti-inflammatory one. Major anti-inflammatory actions are (1) inhibition of migration and accumulation of neutrophils at inflammatory sites through down regulating pro-inflammatory cytokines and adhesion molecules including IL-8 and ICAM-1; (2) inhibition of the epithelial damage by superoxide and elastase from neutrophils and migrating inflammatory cells; (3) inhibition of the hyperseccretion through blocking chloride channel and production of mucin core protein; (4) inhibition of bacterial adherence and biofilm formation.[1,12]

Inhibition of vascular endothelial growth factor production by macrolides

Major pathophysiological activities of the vascular endothelial growth factor (VEGF), identified in 1980s, are angiogenesis and increasing vascular leakage.[13,14] Hypoxia is one of the most effective inducers of VEGF production, and tumor necrosis factor (TNF)-alpha produces the most marked up-regulation of VEGF among all the inflammatory cytokines.[15,16]

By enhancing neovascularization and vasopermeability, VEGF plays an important role in tumor growth, as well as inflammation of the upper and lower respiratory tract. Accordingly, VEGF has been one of the important inflammatory cytokines in chronic airway inflammation. We have reported the importance of VEGF in perpetuating CRS for a number of reasons: (1) increased levels of VEGF are observed in the sinus effusions of patients with CRS compared with VEGF levels within the serum and nasal secretions of these patients, suggesting that VEGF is produced in the paranasal sinus mucosa; (2) hypoxia and increased levels of TNF- alpha are often found in effusions from the paranasal antrum in

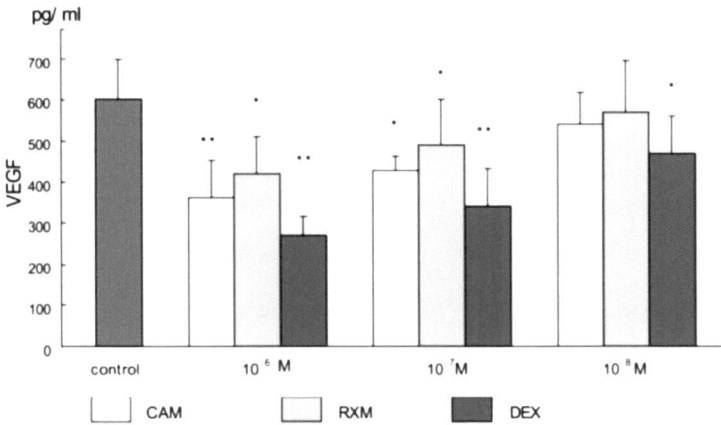

Fig. 3. Vascular endothelial growth factor (VEGF) production was significantly inhibited by exposure to 106 M and 107 M of clarithromycin (CAM), roxithromycin (RXM), or dexamethasone (DEX) during culture under hypoxic conditions for 10 and 20 hours. Only DEX was observed to have an inhibitory effect on VEGF production at a dose of 108 M. CAM had a more marked effect than RXM at 106 M. *P .05; **P .01.

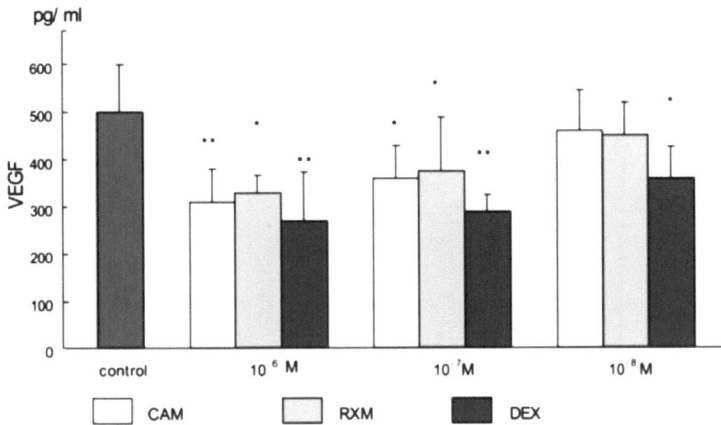

Fig. 4. Vascular endothelial growth factor (VEGF) production was significantly inhibited by exposure to 106 M and 107 M of clarithromycin (CAM), roxithromycin (RXM), or dexamethasone (DEX) during culture with 10 ng/mL tumor necrosis factor for 10 and 20 hours. Only DEX was observed to have an inhibitory effect on VEGF production at a dose of 108 M. CAM had a more marked effect than RXM at 106 M. *P .05; **P .01.

patients with CRS, likely the result of impaired ventilation and drainage between the nasal cavity and paranasal sinuses. In order to study a new mechanism of efficacy of 14-membered ring macrolides in treating CRS, inhibitory effects of macrolides on VEGF production were examined *in vitro*; VEGF production in cultured fibroblasts from human nasal polyps obtained from surgery for CRS stimulated by hypoxia or TNF-alpha was assessed under the administration of CAM or RXM by enzyme linked immunosorbent assay (ELISA) and reverse transcriptase polymerase chain-reaction (RT-PCR). Dose-dependent inhibitory effects on VEGF production stimulated by hypoxia or TNF-alpha were noted in the groups treated with CAM and RXM (Figs. 3 and 4), including inhibition of VEGF mRNA levels. Inhibition of VEGF production was shown to be another important anti-inflammatory mechanism of macrolide in CRS cases.[17-19]

Expectation of successful new 'new macrolide therapy' by EM 900 series in the future

Since macrolide therapy by EM or new macrolides of CAM and RXM has been advocated in the field of upper and lower respiratory inflammation, developing macrolide-resistant bacteria has been mistaken as a possible serious risk. If the anti-inflammatory activity of macrolides is independent of their bactericidal effect, novel anti-inflammatory macrolides without antimicrobial activity should be developed to minimize this kind of risk. In order to achieve this aim EM 700 and EM 900 series have been synthesized as EM derivatives recently, and EM 900 series have been proved to be more effective *in vivo* than EM 700 series. EM 900 series are now regarded as the most promising anti-inflammatory 12-membered lactone ring macrolides without antibiotic activities and a project of innovative drug development is to be kicked off in the near future. EM 900 series are expected to induce new 'new macrolide therapy' for CRS.[20,21]

References

1.   Cervin A, Wallwork B. Macrolide therapy of chronic rhinosinusitis. Rhinology 2007;45:259-267.
2.   Kudoh S, Azuma A, Yamamoto M, et al. Improvement of survival in patients with diffuse panbronchiolitis treated with lowdose erythromycin. Am J Respir Crit Care Med 1998;157:1829-1832.
3.   Keicho N, Kudoh S. Diffuse panbronchiolitis: role of macrolides in therapy. Am J Respir Med 2002;1:119-131.
4.   Kikuchi S, Suzaki H, Aoki A, Ito O, Nomura Y. Clinical effect of long-term low-dose erythromycin therapy for chronic sinusitis Pract Otol (Kyoto) 1991;84;41-47. (In Japanese with English abstract)
5.   Hashiba M, Suzaki H, Furuta S, et al. Guideline for macrolide treatment of chronic paranasal sinusitis (draft). Jpn J Antibiot 1998;51(Suppl A):86-89.
6.   Iino Y, Esawa T, Kobayashi H, et al. Guidelines in macrolide therapy for children with suppurative otitis media]. Jpn J Antibiot 2003;56(Suppl A):167-170.
7.   Ohyama M, Ueno K, Matsune S, et al. Current Status on Macrolide Therapy in Chronic Sinusitis. Pract Otol (Kyoto) 1999;92:571-582. (In Japanese with English abstract)
8.   Pynnonen MA, Venkatraman G, Davis G. Macrolide therapy for chronic rhinosinusitis: A meta-analysis. Otolaryngol Head Neck Surg 2013;148:366-373.
9.   Fokkens WJ, Lund VJ, Mullol J, et al. European position paper on rhinosinusitis and nasal polyps. Rhinology 2012;50(Suppl 23):149-150, 180-181.

10. Wallwork B, Coman W, Mackay-Sim A, Greiff L, Cervin A. A double-blind, randomized, placebo-controlled trial of macrolide in the treatment of chronic rhinosinusitis. Laryngoscope 2006;116:189-193.

11. Yamada T, Fujieda S, Mori S, Yamamoto H, Saito H. Macrolide treatment decreased the size of nasal polyps and IL-8 levels in nasal lavage. Am J Rhinol 2000;14:143-148.

12. Nagaoka K, Yanagihara K, Harada Y, et al. Macrolides inhibit Fusobacterium nucleatum-induced MUC5AC production in human airway epithelial cells. Antimicrob Agents Chemother 2013;57:1844-1849.

13. Ferrara N, Henzel WJ. Pituitary follicular cells secrete anovel heparin-binding growth factor specific for vascular endothelial cells. BiochemBiophys Res Commun 1989;161:851-858.

14. Senger D, Galli SJ, Dvorak AM, et al. Tumor cells secrete a vascular permeability factor which promotes ascites fluid accumulation. Science 1983;219:983-985.

15. Shweiki D, Itin A, Soffer D, et al. Vascular endothelial growth factor induced by hypoxia may mediate hypoxia-initiated angiogenesis. Nature 1992;359:843-845.

16. Bottomley MJ, Webb NJA, Watson CJ, et al. Peripheral blood mononuclear cells from patients with rheumatoid arthritis spontaneously secrete vascular endothelial growth factor (VEGF): specific up-regulation by tumor necrosis factor-alpha (TNF-) in synovial fluid. Clin Exp Immunol 1999;117:171-176.

17. Matsune S, Kono M, Sun D, et al. Hypoxia in paranasal sinuses of patients with chronic sinusitis with or without the complication of nasal allergy. Acta Otolaryngol 2003;123:519-523.

18. Sun D, Matsune S, Ohori J, et al. TNF- and endotoxin increase hypoxia-induced VEGF production by cultured human nasal fibroblasts in synergistic fashion. Auris Nasus Larynx 2005;32:243-249.

19. Matsune S, Sun D, Ohori J, et al. Inhibition of vascular endothelial growth factor by macrolides in cultured fibroblasts from nasal polyps. Laryngoscope 2005;115:1953-1956.

20. Otsu K, Ishinaga H, Suzuki S, et al. Effects of a novel nonantibiotic macrolide, EM900, on cytokine and mucin gene expression in a human airway epithelial cell line. Pharmacology 2011;88:327-332.

21. Sugawara A, Sueki A, Hirose T, et al. Novel 12-membered non-antibiotic macrolides from erythromycin A; EM900 series as novel leads for anti-inflammatory and/or immunomodulatory agents. Bioorg Med Chem Lett 2011;21:3373-3376.

RHINOSINUSITIS WITH PROLONGED COUGH IN CHILDREN

S. Masuda

Department of Otorhinolaryngology, National Mie Hospital, Mie, Japan

Introduction

Cough is one of the most frequent symptoms in children. A survey[1] about prevalence of respiratory symptoms in Japanese preschool children based on a nationwide mail questionnaire showed that 94.8% of children had experienced nasal symptoms in a recent year, followed by nonproductive cough or wet cough. However, sometimes the diagnosis and proper treatment to the disease causing the cough was delayed.

Rhinosinusitis is found frequently in children with chronic cough. According to Tatli,[2] sinus abnormality on the CT scan was found in 66.7% of 42 children with cough lasting for more than four weeks.

I herein report the case of a child who had been suffering from prolonged cough caused by rhinosinusitis.

Case report

A four-year-old boy was complaining of prolonged cough. He had been coughing since 13 months ago. The cough was productive, occurring without any triggers. His mother noticed neither his nasal symptoms, nor wheezing.

He was diagnosed with bronchial asthma and treated with leukotriene antagonists and inhaled corticosteroids. He visited our pediatric department for a detailed examination of asthma. The pediatrician introduced him to us.

In his nasal cavity, there was mucopurulent nasal discharge. The inferior turbinate was swollen and the middle nasal meatus was blocked. The dominant inflammatory cells in nasal secretion were neutrophils. Serum IgE specific to

Address for correspondence: Sawako Masuda, MD, Department of Otorhinolaryngology, National Mie Hospital , 357 Osato-Kubota, Tsu, Mie 514-0125, Japan. E-mail: masudas@mie-m.hosp.go.jp

Recent Advances in Rhinosinusitis and Nasal Polyposis, pp. 147-150
Edited by Hideyuki Kawauchi, Desiderio Passali, Ranko Mladina, Andrey Lopatin and Dmytro Zabolotnyi
2015 © Kugler Publications, Amsterdam, The Netherlands

house dust mite, Japanese cedar, cat, and dog were all negative. Waters' view X-ray revealed soft tissue density in the right maxillary sinus. Finally, he was diagnosed with rhinosinusitis.

He was treated with clarithromycin at a dose of five mg per kilogram per day. All medicines for asthma were stopped. We advised him to practice blowing the nose. The cough decreased in one week, and disappeared in three weeks.

Rhinosinusitis and prolonged cough

Rhinosinusitis is one of the important causes of coughing, however, it is often overlooked, under-diagnosed or misdiagnosed as in this case. Therefore, we investigated 32 children (17 boys and 15 girls, one-15 years of age, the median age was four) presenting with cough lasting for more than four weeks.[3] Pediatricians and otorhinolaryngologists examined each patient on the same day. A questionnaire was filled out by their parents.

Figure 1 shows the combination of diagnoses by pediatricians and otorhinolaryngologists. The disease most frequently diagnosed by pediatricians was asthma. Some patients had bronchitis, psychogenic cough, pneumonia, or whooping cough. In 34% of the subjects, no problems were found in the pediatric department. On the other hand, in the ENT department, 50% and 44% of the children were diagnosed with sinusitis and allergic rhinitis, respectively. All the children with sinusitis had productive or mixed-type cough. Most of the children with allergic rhinitis also had asthma. A few of the patients with rhinosinusitis had bronchitis or asthma.

Type of cough: ▲Productive □Mixed ●Dry

		Otorhinolaryngological diagnosis			
		Sinusitis (11)	Sinusitis and allergic rhinitis(5)	Allergic rhinitis (9)	None (7)
Pediatric diagnosis	Asthma (13)	▲		▲▲▲ ●●●●●	▲▲□●
	Bronchitis (5)	▲	□□□		▲
	Psychogenic cough (2)				●●
	Whooping cough (1)			●	
	None (11)	▲▲▲▲▲ ▲▲▲▲	▲▲		

Fig. 1. Combination of diagnoses by otorhinolaryngologist and pediatrician in 32 children with prolonged cough.

Eighty-eight percent of the children with rhinosinusitis were treated with clarithromycin, 14-membered macrolide, in a dose of 5-7 mg/kg/day. After a month of treatment, 57% of them cured, 25% improved, 6% partially improved. That is, appropriate treatment for a month resulted in significant improvement in more than 80% of the children with cough caused by chronic rhinosinusitis.

Primary ciliary dyskinesia

However, sometimes rhinosinusitis is intractable in spite of treatments. Primary ciliary dyskinesia (PCD) is not frequently diagnosed but it is one of the important diseases in children with intractable chronic rhinosinusitis and prolonged productive cough. Abnormality of ciliary structure and function resulting from autosomal recessive disorder causes various clinical symptoms. The symptoms include chronic airway infections, such as sinusitis and otitis media with effusion. *Situs inversus* is seen in half the patients, and it is well known as Kartagener's syndrome.

Diagnosis of PCD is sometimes difficult, especially in the patients without *situs inversus*. PCD should be suspected when the patient has symmetric respiratory diseases, both upper and lower airway involvement, including middle ears. Chin et al.[4] described that the presence of multiple clinical manifestations (sinonasal, otitis media, and/or pulmonary) is a good predictor of PCD. In the newborn period, continuous rhinorrhea from the first day of life is observed. In childhood, chronic productive cough, rhinosinusitis, and otitis media are important findings[5] for otorhinolaryngologists. However, nasal polyps are not so frequently found in the patients with PCD.[6]

One of the hints for diagnosis is small frontal and sphenoid sinuses.[6] Pifferi et al.[7] reported that more than half of patients have aplastic or hypoplastic frontal and/or sphenoid sinuses. Another important finding in PCD patients is decreased production of nasal nitric oxide (NO).[8] The measurement of nasal NO is a valuable tool for the screening of PCD. Other manifestations are persistent otitis media with effusion and prolonged wet cough. The combination of these diseases is important. The diagnostic process of PCD is shown in Figure 2. Characteristic clinical phenotype is important, nasal NO measurement is helpful as screening, and electron microscopy and/or genetic examination confirm the diagnosis.

Conclusion

A rhinological approach is important to evaluate and manage prolonged cough in pediatric patients. We should pay attention to a rare disease such as PCD.

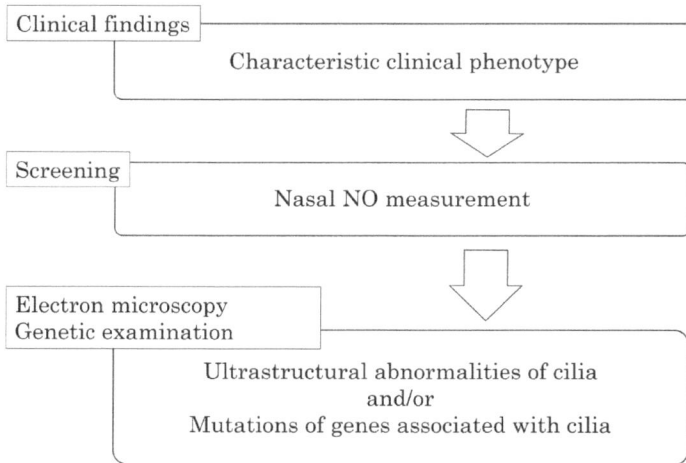

Fig. 2. Diagnostic process of PCD.

Acknowledgement

I am grateful to Prof. Kazuhiko Takeuchi for valuable comments and suggestions.

References

1. Mochizuki H, Fujisawa T. Reality of respiratory symptoms in preschool-age children – result of a parental questionnaire. Arerugi 2008;57:1166-1174.
2. Tatli MM, San I, Karaoglanoglu M. Paranasal sinus computed tomographic findings of children with chronic cough. Int J Pediatr Otorhinolaryngol 2001;60:213-217.
3. Masuda S, Fujisawa T, Usui S, et al. Interdisciplinary approach to prolonged cough in children. Shyoniji 2007;28:24-30. [In Japanese.]
4. Chin GY, Karas DE, Kashgarian M. Correlation of presentation and pathologic condition in primary ciliary dyskinesia. Arch Otolaryngol Head Neck Surg 2002;128:1292-1294.
5. Bush A, Chodhari R, Collins N, et al. Primary ciliary dyskinesia: current state of the art. Arch Dis Child 2007;92:1136-1140.
6. Barbato A, Frischer T, Kuehni CE, et al. Primary ciliary dyskinesia: a consensus statement on diagnostic and treatment approaches in children. Eur Respir J 2009;34:1264-1276.
7. Pifferi M, Bush A, Caramella D, et al. Agenesis of paranasal sinuses and nasal nitric oxide in primary ciliary dyskinesia. Eur Respir J 2011;37:566-571.
8. Noone PG, Leigh MW, Sannuti A, et al. Primary ciliary dyskinesia: diagnostic and phenotypic features. Am J Respir Crit Care 2004;169:459-467.

NEUTROPHILS WITH TRIGGERING RECEPTOR EXPRESSED ON MYELOID CELLS (TREM)-1 EXPRESSION ENHANCE BACTERIAL CLEARANCE FROM THE NOSE IN C3H/HEN MICE MORE THAN IN C3H/HEJ MICE

Takashi Hirano, Munehito Moriyama, Toshiaki Kawano, Yoshinori Kadowaki, Taro Iwasaki, Satoru Kodama, Masashi Suzuki

Oita University, Faculty of Medicine, Department of Otolaryngology

Introduction

Chronic rhinosinusitis is a common inflammatory disease of the sinonasal cavity and recent molecular studies have confirmed that *Streptococcus pneumoniae* and non-typeable *Haemophilus influenzae* (NTHi) is important in chronic rhinosinusitis. We investigated the role of toll-like receptor-4 (TLR-4) and triggering receptor expressed on myeloid cells-1 (TREM-1) expression on neutrophil to enhance bacterial clearance from the nose.

The TREM-1 is an activating receptor expressed on neutrophils and monocytes. Engagement of TREM-1 on the surface of the cell membrane leads to activation of a cascade of intracellular events, and results in inflammatory effects, such as cytokine production, degranulation of neutrophils and phagocytosis.[1-3] The ligands of TREM-1 are unclear, although several putative ligands have been proposed, for example platelets, HMGB1, HSP70, peptideglycan, endotoxin.[4] To date, 12 TLRs have been identified in mammals, and TLR-4 are important receptors to induce innate immune responses in the NTHi infection.[5] Also it is reported that biological effects of TREM-1 are suggested to interact with the TLR-4/LPS-receptor complex.[6] In this study, we used C3H/HeJ (TLR-4 mutant mice) and C3H/HeN (wild tipe mice), and we investigate the interaction of TLR-4 and TREM-1 expression by using a nasopharyngeal clearance model in mice.

Address for correspondence: Dr. Takashi Hirano, Oita University, Faculty of Medicine, Department of otolaryngology, 1-1 Idaigaoka, Hasama-machi, Yufu, Oita, Japan, 8795593. Tel: +81-97-586-5913. Fax:+81-97-549-0762. E-mail: thirano@oita-u.ac.jp

Recent Advances in Rhinosinusitis and Nasal Polyposis, pp. 151-154
Edited by Hideyuki Kawauchi, Desiderio Passali, Ranko Mladina, Andrey Lopatin
and Dmytro Zabolotnyi
2015 © Kugler Publications, Amsterdam, The Netherlands

Materials and methods

Animals

C3H/HeJ (TLR-4-mutant) and C3H/HeN (WT) mice were purchased from Charles River Laboratories (Atsugi, Japan). All mice were maintained in a pathogen-free facility until they were six weeks old, at which time they were used.

Bacterial challenge and collecting samples

NTHi (strain 76) isolated in our clinic from the nasopharynx of patients with OME were used. An aliquot of the stored bacteria was cultured on chocolate or blood agar plates overnight at 37°C with 5% CO_2, and suspended in Phosphate buffered saline (PBS) to a concentration of 10^9 CFU/ml. Three mice were intra-nasally injected with 10 μl of NTHi suspension. The animals were decapitated at 12 hours after the challenge with 0.1 mL of 2% ketamine and 0.2% xylazine given intraperitoneally. Nasal washes were collected by irrigation of the naso-pharynx with 200 μl PBS, and bacterial colonies were counted. Nasal mucosae were collected and treated with collagenase type IV for collecting neutrophil in the nasal mucosa to separate single cells. To investigate the expression of TLR-4 on neutrophil in the nasal mucosa, a suspension of single cells was stained with FITC-conjugated anti-Ly-6G monoclonal antibodies (mAb; Beckman Coulter, Fullerton, CA, USA) and PE-conjugated anti-TREM-1 mAb (R&D Systems, Inc., Minneapolis, MN, USA).

Statistics

The Mann-Whitney U test was used to determine the significance of the dif-ferences in the numbers of bacteria cultured from nasal washes. A difference at p < 0.05 was considered significant.

Results

Nasal washes at 12 hours after bacterial challenge in C3H/HeN mice showed a significant reduction in the numbers of bacteria when compared to C3H/HeJ mice. The mean CFU/mL in the C3H/HeN vs. C3H/HeJ challenged at 12 hours after the challenge, 2950 vs. 10700, respectively ($P < 0.05$). At 12 hours after the bacterial challenge, a TREM-1 expression was augmented more in both of two strains. In C3H/HeN mice, cells positive for both TREM-1 and Ly-6G (double-positive) were 52.1% of the nuetrophils. On the other hand, in C3H/HeJ mice, double-positive cells increased up to 40.6% at 12 hours after the bacterial challenge. The percentage of double positive cells was higher in C3H/HeN mice than in C3H/HeJ mice.

Discussion

Activation and expression of TREM-1 by neutrophils occurs in concert with TLR-4 for bacterial lipopolysaccharide. It is reported that using pharmacological inhibitors and western blot analysis, phosphatidyl inositide 3-kinase, phospholipase C and the mitogen-activated kinase p38MAPK are essential for the TREM-1- and TLR-4-induced oxidative burst of human PMN.[6] In this study, we sought to investigate the putative effects of TREM-1 activation in neutrophils in relation with NTHi challenge and TLR-4. NTHi clearance from the nose augmented significantly in C3H/HeN mice when compared to C3H/HeJ mice at 12 hours after bacterial challenge, and TREM-1 expression on neutrophil in the nasal mucosa also increased in C3H/HeN mice when compared to C3H/HeJ mice. Our results also showed the TREM-1 interaction with the LPS/TLR-4 receptor complex in the upper airway inflammation with NTHi, including the nasopharynx. It is reported that engagement of TREM-1 can exert beneficial effects through the activation of antibacterial host defense, as shown in an experimental model of pneumonia.[7] In future, TREM-1 stimulation may be a new strategy for bacterial infection in the upper airway.

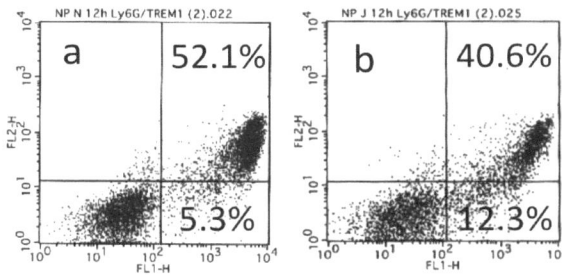

Fig. 1. In C3H/HeN mice, the cells positive for both TREM-1 and Ly-6G (double-positive) were 52.1% of the neutrophils. On the other hand, in C3H/HeJ mice, double-positive cells increased up to 40.6% at 12 hours after the bacterial challenge.

References

1. Bouchon A, Dietrich J, Colonna M. Cutting edge: Inflammatory responses can be triggered by TREM-1, a novel receptor expressed on neutrophils and monocytes. J Immunol 2000;164:4991-4995.
2. Radsak MP, Salih HR, Rammensee HG, Schild H. Triggering receptor expressed on myeloid cells-1 in neutrophil inflammatory responses: Differential regulation of activation and survival. J Immunol 2004;172:4956-4963.
3. Haselmayer P, Grosse-Hovest L, von Landenberg P, Schild H, Radsak MP. TREM-1 ligand expression on platelets enhances neutrophil activation. Blood 2007;110:1029-1035.
4. Arts RJ, Joosten LA, van der Meer JW, Netea MG. TREM-1: intracellular signaling pathways and interaction with pattern recognition receptors. J Leukoc Biol 2013;93:209-215.

5. Hirano T, Kodama S, Fujita K, Maeda K, Suzuki M. Role of Toll-like receptor 4 in innate immune responses in a mouse model of acute otitis media. FEMS Immunol Med Microbiol 2007;49:75-83.
6. Haselmayer P, Daniel M, Tertilt C, Salih HR, Stassen M,et al. Signaling pathways of the TREM-1- and TLR4-mediated neutrophil oxidative burst. J Innate Immun 2009;1:582-591.
7. Lagler H, Sharif O, Haslinger I, Matt U, Stich K, et al. TREM-1 activation alters the dynamics of pulmonary IRAK-M expression in vivo and improves host defense during pneumococcal pneumonia. J Immunol 2009;183:2027-2036.

MUCOSAL IMMUNOGLOBULIN E-POSITIVE CELLS IN CASES OF CHRONIC RHINOSINUSITIS WITH ASTHMA

Yasushi Ota[1], Yoshihiro Ikemiyagi[1], Mutsunori Fujiwara[2], Toshio Kumasaka[3], Tamiko Takemura[3], Mitsuya Suzuki[1]

[1]Department of Otorhinolaryngology Toho University Sakura Medical Center, Chiba, Japan, [2]Department of Clinical Laboratory Japanese Red Cross Medical Center, Tokyo, Japan, [3]Department of Pathology Japanese Red Cross Medical Center, Tokyo, Japan

Abstract

Background: Chronic rhinosinusitis (CRS) is often complicated with asthma. An anti-immunoglobulin (Ig) E antibody has shown efficacy in the treatment of CRS and asthma, but the underlying mechanisms are not fully understood.
Objective: To investigate the relationship between IgE-positive cell-containing mucosal lymphoid follicles, eosinophils, and asthma-related complications in Japanese CRS patients.
Methods: Participants were 19 Japanese CRS patients who attended the Japanese Red Cross Medical Centre Otorhinolaryngology Department between July 2011 and August 2012. Paranasal sinus mucosa samples were obtained and stained with hematoxylin and eosin (HE) and immunostained with anti-IgE antibody. The number of IgE-positive cells and eosinophils was counted both in the circulation and in tissues. The presence of lymphoid follicles was determined on paranasal sinus mucosa tissue sections.
Results: Asthma was diagnosed in ten of the 19 patients. The number of IgE-positive cells and eosinophils in the paranasal sinus mucosa was significantly higher in the patients with asthma than in those without asthma (p = 0.00024 and p = 0.00044, respectively). The circulating eosinophil count and total IgE level

Address for correspondence: Yasushi Ota, Department of Otorhinolaryngology, Toho University Sakura Medical Center, 564-1 Shimoshizu Sakura, Chiba 285-8741, Japan.
E-mail: takashi160112@yahoo.co.jp

Recent Advances in Rhinosinusitis and Nasal Polyposis, pp. 155-164
Edited by Hideyuki Kawauchi, Desiderio Passali, Ranko Mladina, Andrey Lopatin
and Dmytro Zabolotnyi
2015 © Kugler Publications, Amsterdam, The Netherlands

were also significantly higher in patients with asthma than in those without asthma (p = 0.00024 and p = 0.00136, respectively). Relapse of CRS was observed one year postoperatively in patients with asthma but not in patients without asthma. Five of the ten CRS with asthma exhibited intramucosal lymphoid follicles, which stained strongly for the IgE and the B-cell marker CD20. None of CRS patients without asthma showed presence of intramucosal lymphoid follicles.

Conclusions: The localized production of large quantities of IgE by the paranasal sinus mucosa might induce infiltration of the mucosa by eosinophils. This mechanism is thought to result in the intractability and relapse of rhinosinusitis observed in eosinophilic CRS patients.

Keywords: asthma, eosinophilic rhinosinusitis, endoscopic sinus surgery, eosinophil, lymphoid follicles, paranasal mucosa

Introduction

The use of transnasal endoscopic surgery, also known as endoscopic sinus surgery, for the treatment of chronic rhinosinusitis (CRS) has gained popularity in Japan in the latter half of the 1980s. In the early 1990s, low-dose long-term treatment with erythromycin (EM) was established.[1,2] Endoscopic sinus surgery enables restoration of ventilation while preserving the sinus mucosa, and low-dose long-term EM treatment helps normalization of the residual mucosa.

Since the latter half of the 1990s, however, the incidence of intractable relapsing CRS due to resistance to low-dose long-term EM therapy increased. Cases of intractable relapsing CRS are characterized by increased number of eosinophils both in circulation and in tissues as well as by an extremely high rate of asthma-related complications. In 2001, Haruna *et al.* proposed the concept of 'eosinophilic CRS' for this type of sinusitis.[3] Thereafter, while the cause and curative treatment for eosinophilic CRS remained to be elucidated, the number of patients suffering from the condition tended to increase.

Eosinophilic CRS is frequently complicated with asthma, is highly intractable, and relapses relatively early following paranasal sinus surgery. It is characterized by an increase in the number of circulating peripheral eosinophils, with marked eosinophilic infiltration of the paranasal sinus mucosa. Systemic administration of steroids is an effective treatment, but long-term therapy cannot be continued because of its side effects. Thus, currently, there is no definitive treatment for this condition. Treatment involves a combination of surgery, antihistamines, anti-leukotrienes, and steroid sprays, but these treatment approaches have limitations, and a large number of patients experience recurrent episodes of remission and relapse.

Immunoglobulin (Ig) E is produced by plasma cells and binds to mast cells, resulting in the production of various cytokines. Some of these cytokines, such as RANTES, eotaxin, interleukin- (IL-)5, and intercellular adhesion molecule-

(ICAM-)1, are involved in eosinophilic migration and adhesion, causing eosinophilic infiltration. The presence of excess IgE in allergic fungal sinusitis, considered as one type of eosinophilic CRS, has already been reported.[4] Interestingly, the anti-IgE antibody, omalizumab, has been reported to effectively treat eosinophilic CRS and eosinophilic tympanitis, implicating IgE as a cause of the eosinophilic infiltrate in eosinophilic CRS.[5,6] However, the underlying mechanisms are not yet fully understood.

Tsurumaru[7] reported the existence of lymphoid follicles that function first-line defense structures in the sinus mucosa of CRS patients. In this study, we investigated the relationship between IgE-positive cell-containing mucosal lymphoid follicles, eosinophils, and asthma-related complications in Japanese CRS patients.

Patients and methods

Participants were 19 patients (eight males, 11 females) who attended the Japanese Red Cross Medical Center Otorhinolaryngology Department between July 2011 and August 2012. The median patient age was 45.5 years (range: 14-76 years).

Subjects were selected from among patients with CRS who had undergone endoscopic sinus surgery. For each patient, we evaluated the clinical characteristics, lower respiratory tract disease, postoperative paranasal sinus mucosal hypertrophy, intramucosal lymphoid follicles, and circulating IgE, tissue levels of IgE-positive cells, circulating eosinophils % and tissue levels of eosinophils.

Paranasal sinus mucosa specimens obtained from the subjects were fixed in neutral buffered formalin solution and then were embedded in paraffin, after which they were sectioned. Next, immunohistochemical staining was performed using the ABC method with PA1-29206 rabbit anti-human IgE antibody (Thermo Scientific, Rockford, USA) as the primary antibody. Then, hematoxylin and eosin (HE) staining was performed.

The degree of infiltration by IgE-positive cells and eosinophils was assessed using the method established by Sakuma's laboratory.[8] Briefly, the number of IgE-positive cells and eosinophils was counted in five optical fields (magnification: 400 x). For each specimen, the three fields with the highest cell counts were used to calculate the mean number of infiltrating IgE-positive cells and eosinophils.

The presence of intramucosal lymphoid follicles was investigated using the same paranasal sinus mucosa histopathological preparations.

Circulating IgE, intramucosal IgE-positive cells, circulating eosinophils % and eosinophil cell counts were compared between CRS patients with and without concurrent asthma and between CRS patients concurrent asthma with and without intramucosal lymphoid folliclesby using Mann-Whitney's U-test.

Results

The clinical characteristics of the 19 CRS patients are shown in Table 1. Asthma was diagnosed in ten of the 19 patients.

Table 1. Clinical profiles of the 19 patients in this study

	Lymphoid follicles	Tissue IgE count	Circulating total IgE (µg/ml)	Tissue eosinophil count	Circulating eosinophil count (%)	Lower respiratory tract disease	Postoperative paranasal sin mucosal hypertrophy
36F	+	85	64	86	6.8	Asthma for 5 years	Mild
46F	+	68.7	123	70	12.8	Asthma for 5 years	None
23F	+	57.3	245	57	21.6	Asthma since child-hood	Severe
33F	+	86	327	78	9.9	Asthma for 3 years	Mild
57F	+	62.7	2204	51	9.4	Asthma for 12 years	Moderate
55F	−	59.7	64	37	11.3	Asthma for 12 years	Mild
40M	−	114	90	110	12.4	Asthma for 5 years	Severe
31M	−	76.3	232	257	11.2	Asthma since child-hood	Severe
63M	−	166.3	139	7	10.4	Asthma for 4 years	Severe
33M	−	76.7	186	130	11.2	Asthma since child-hood	Severe
39 F	−	13.3	8	34.7	4.6	None	None
14M	−	22.7	52	4.7	4.2	None	None
57M	−	18.3		6	3.8	None	None
41M	−	29	80	2.3	3	None	None
74M	−	27.7	72	4.7	1.8	None	None
23M	−	13.3	11	3	0.4	None	None
60M	−	16	8	27.3	2.9	None	None
63M	−	8.3	33	6.3	4.5	None	None
76F	−	4	41	4.7	1.6	None	None

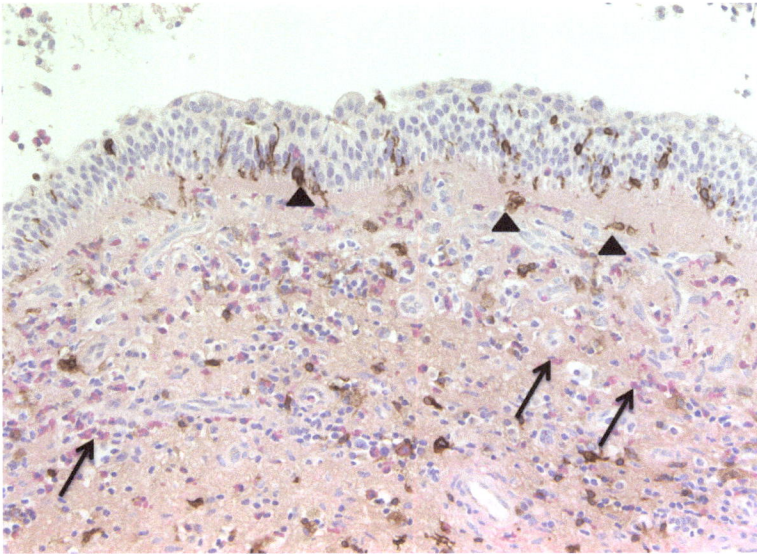

Fig. 1. Infiltration of IgE-positive cells and eosinophils in the paranasal sinus mucosa of a patient with CRS and asthma. Several IgE-positive cells and eosinophils are observed in the mucosa. Arrows, eosinophils; arrowheads, IgE-positive cells. Magnification: 20 × 10.

A large number of IgE-positive cells and eosinophils was observed in the paranasal sinus mucosa of the 10 CRS patients with concurrent asthma (Fig. 1). On the other hand, few or no IgE-positive cells and eosinophils infiltrated the paranasal sinus mucosa of the 9 CRS patients without concurrent asthma (Fig. 2). Cell counts revealed that the number of IgE-positive cells and eosinophils in the paranasal sinus mucosa was indeed significantly higher in patients with asthma than in those without asthma (IgE-positive cell count: 82.1 versus 15.8 [p = 0.00024] and eosinophil cell count: 88 versus 10.4 [p = 0.00044], respectively; Fig. 3).

The circulating eosinophil % (total white blood cell count: 11.7% versus 2.3%, respectively [p = 0.00024]) as well as the mean circulating total IgE level (401.5 µl/ml versus 33.8 µl/ml, respectively [p = 0.00136]) was significantly higher in patients with asthma than in those without asthma. The circulating eosinophil % and circulating total IgE in patients without asthma were within the normal range. However, in the 10 CRS patients with concurrent asthma, circulating total IgE level was 64-2204 µg/ml, ranging from normal to markedly elevated.

Approximately one year postoperatively, relapse was observed in the ten CRS patients with asthma but not in the nine CRS patients without asthma (data not shown).

Histopathological analysis revealed the presence of intramucosal lymphoid follicles in five of the ten CRS patients with concurrent asthma. Photographs of a typical intramucosal lymphoid follicle are shown in Figure 4. All observed

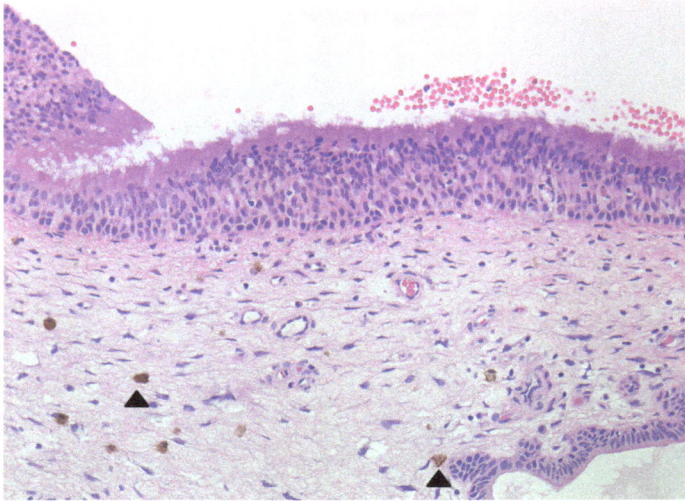

Fig. 2. Paranasal sinus mucosa of a patient with CRS but no concurrent asthma. A few IgE-positive cells and almost no eosinophils are observed in the mucosa. Arrowheads, IgE-positive cells. Magnification: 20 × 10.

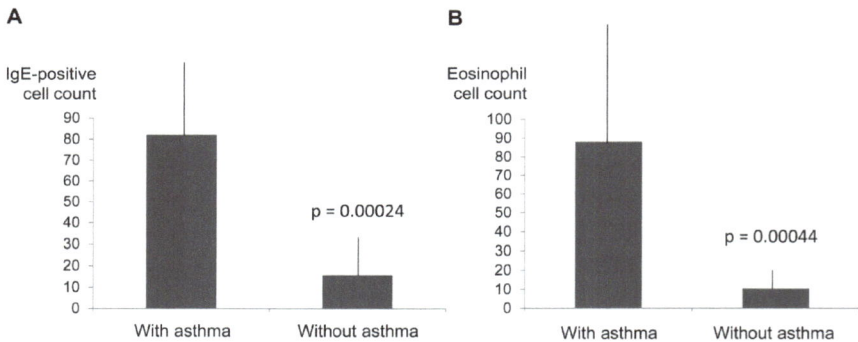

Fig. 3. Intramucosal IgE-positive cells and eosinophils in CRS patients with and without asthma. A significant difference in (A) IgE-positive cell count and (B) eosinophil count was observed between patients with and without asthma. Results are expressed as mean ± standard deviation.

intramucosal lymphoid follicles were stained strongly with anti-IgE antibody. The presence of germinal centers was also observed. The cells infiltrated into the intramucosal lymphoid follicles were not stained with an anti-CD3 antibody but stained positive for CD20 (L26), indicating the presence of B lymphocytes (Fig. 5).

The average number of paranasal sinus mucosal IgE-positive cells in the five CRS patients with concurrentt asthma and intramucosal lymphoid follicles was 71.9, and the average eosinophil count was 68.4, while in the remaining five cases (where no intramucosal lymphoid follicles were observed), the average

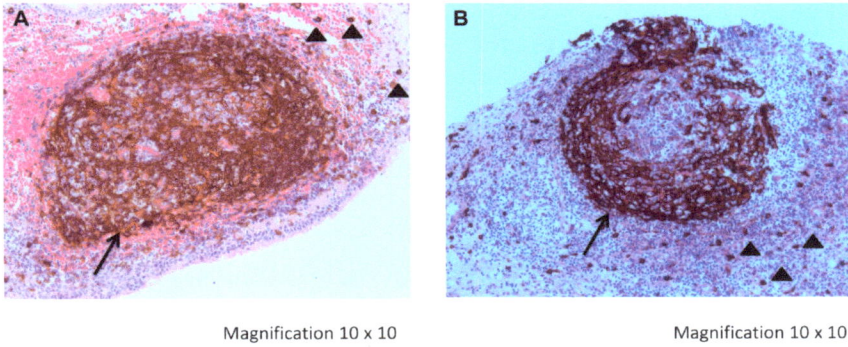

Magnification 10 x 10   Magnification 10 x 10

Fig. 4. Nasal mucosa-associated lymphoid follicles in CRS patients with concurrent asthma. Shown are two representative images (A and B). Arrows, lymphoid tissue, where IgE-positive cells have accumulated, with visible germinal center; arrowheads, IgE-positive cells.

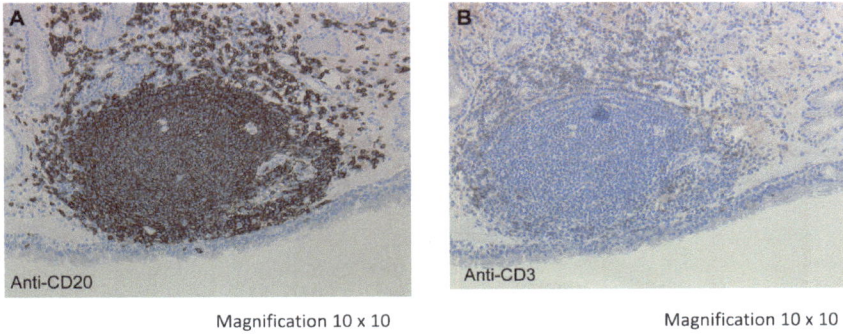

Anti-CD20   Anti-CD3

Magnification 10 x 10   Magnification 10 x 10

Fig. 5. B cells and T cells in the lymphoid follicles. (A) B-cell marker anti-CD20 (anti-L26) antibody stained B lymphocytes as well as large areas of the lymphoid follicles. (B) Anti-CD3 antibody stained T lymphocytes but not the lymphoid follicle cells.

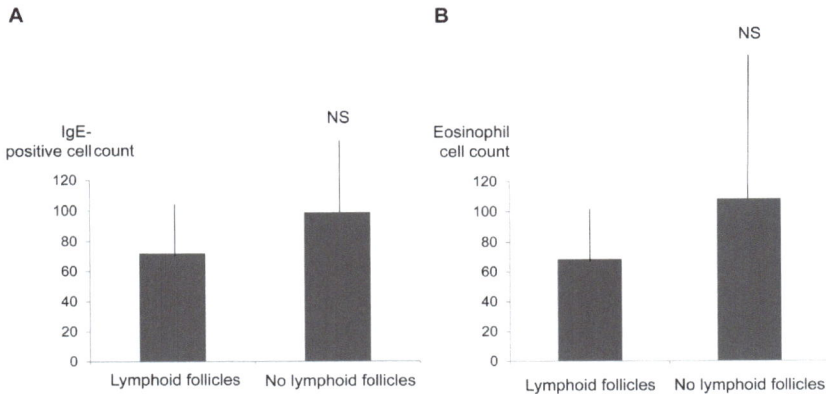

Fig. 6. Infiltration of IgE-positive cells and eosinophils in the paranasal sinus mucosa according to the presence or absence of lymphoid follicles. No statistically significant difference in (A) IgE-positive cell count and (B) eosinophil count was observed between patients with and without lymphoid follicles. NS, not significant. Results are expressed as mean ± standard deviation.

number of mucosal IgE-positive cells was 98.6, with an average eosinophil count of 108.2. These differences were not significantly different (Fig. 6).

In the 9 CRS patients without concurrent asthma, no lymphoid follicles were found in the paranasal sinus mucosa.

Discussion

Chronic rhinosinusitis with nasal polyps and allergic rhinitis is characterized by Th2 inflammatory responses, eosinophilia, and IgE synthesis.[5] We investigated the relationship between IgE, eosinophils, and asthma-related complications in Japanese CRS patients.

In our series, none of the patients without asthma had relapse of CRS after surgery. In contrast, postoperative relapse of CRS occurred in all ten patients with concurrent asthma. This suggests an obvious difference in paranasal mucosal histology between patients with and without concurrent asthma.

In this study, the CRS patients with concurrent asthma had high IgE values and IgE-positive cell and eosinophil counts both in the paranasal mucosa and in circulation. These patients presented with clinically intractable and relapsing CRS, in line with the definition of eosinophilic CRS. The CRS patients without concurrent asthma had low IgE values and IgE-positive cell and eosinophil counts in the paranasal mucosa and in circulation. These patients achieved control status easily in terms of their clinical symptoms of CRS, and their condition was classified as infective CRS.

Matsuwaki *et al.*[9] reported that patients with a high total peripheral eosinophil count and those with asthma were likely to experience recurrence of CRS within five years after surgery. This is consistent with our results.

Tsurumaru[7] reported the presence of intramucosal lymphoid follicles in the maxillary sinus mucosa in 14 of 27 CRS cases. These intramucosal lymphoid follicles are thought to participate in mucosal inflammation.

The stroma of the normal paranasal sinus mucosa contains lymphocytes and plasma cells, but no lymphoid aggregates.[10,11]

In this report, intramucosal lymphoid follicles were found in five of ten CRS cases with concurrent asthma, and all follicles were strongly stained by an anti-IgE antibody. The intramucosal lymphoid follicles in cases of CRS with concurrent asthma are thought to participate heavily in intramucosal IgE production. These intramucosal lymphoid follicles are also conjectured to arise due to the aggregation of B lymphocytes. Irrespective of the presence or absence of intramucosal lymphoid follicles, the ten CRS cases with concurrent asthma showed high levels of infiltration by IgE-positive cells and eosinophils in the paranasal sinus mucosa. The average number of paranasal sinus mucosal IgE-positive cells and eosinophils was not significantly different between patients with and without lymphoid follicles. This observation suggests the presence of similar pathological changes in the paranasal sinus mucosa in CRS with concurrent asthma both with and without lymphoid follicles.

Because paranasal sinus surgery was conducted via intranasal endoscopy in all cases, normal paranasal mucosa was preserved. In addition, only small excised mucosal specimens were examined histopathologically. Therefore, it is possible that IgE-positive intramucosal lymphoid follicles might exist in almost all cases of CRS with concurrent asthma that have abnormal sinus mucosa.

No intramucosal lymphoid follicles were observed in the mucosa of CRS cases without concurrent asthma. According to previous reports,[7] these cases are also thought to form intramucosal lymphoid follicles, but the frequency compared to cases with concurrent asthma is low. Thus, it is believed that lymphoid follicles were simply not included in the excised pathology specimens.

As mentioned above, the anti-IgE antibody, omalizumab, has been reported to effectively treat eosinophilic CRS.[5,6] Djukanovic et al. reported that treatment with omalizumab resulted in marked reduction serum IgE levels and numbers of IgE-positive cells in the airway mucosa; tissue eosinophils; cells positive for the high-affinity Fc receptor for IgE; CD3-positive, CD4-positive, and CD8-negative T lymphocytes; B lymphocytes; and cells stained for IL4.[12] Massanari et al. reported that peripheral blood eosinophil counts were significantly reduced from baseline in omalizumab-treated patients but not in the placebo group.[13] From these facts, IgE is thought to be related to eosinophilic inflammation.

The life span of antibody-producing cells is generally short (around two weeks), and the circulating half-life of IgE is even shorter (around one day).[14] In addition, although there were secondary follicles with germinal centers in some of the intramucosal lymphoid follicles that were observed in the cases of CRS with concurrent asthma, continuous antigen stimulation is said to be required for the formation and maintenance of secondary follicles in lymphoid tissue.[15]

Gevaert et al.[16] reported that the organization of secondary lymphoid tissue with IgE in polyp tissue and a polyclonal hyper-immunoglobulinemia E was associated with the presence of IgE antibodies to Staphylococcus aureus enterotoxins, colonization with S. aureus, and tissue eosinophilia in a relevant subgroup of polyp patients. Bachert et al.[17] reported that because the use of anti-IgE antibodies is a valid treatment approach for nasal polyps and comorbid asthma in atopic and nonatopic patients, S. aureus enterotoxin-IgE-associated polyclonal IgE is functional.

Based on these facts, continuous exposure to an antigen and continuous IgE production is thought to be required for the formation of intractable, relapsing pathological changes found in CRS. The continuous localized production of IgE in the paranasal sinus mucosa induces infiltration of eosinophils to the mucosa and is thought to lead the formation of the intractable pathology found in eosinophilic CRS, that is different from traditional infective CRS.

Conclusion

The large number of eosinophils that infiltrate into the paranasal mucosa in CRS with concurrent asthma is thought to be the response to the production of large quantities of IgE by intramucosal lymphoid follicles. This is thought to result in intractability and relapse of CRS observed in eosinophilic CRS patients.

Conflicts of interest

The authors declare no conflicts of interest.

References

1. Suzaki H, Kikuchi S, Ibuki S. Administration of low-dose long-term erythromycin as treatment for chronic paranasal sinusitis. Effects against inflammatory cytokines. Ther Res 1994;15:4733-4734.
2. Kikuchi S, Yamasoba T, Suzaki H. Paranasal sinusitis and administration of low-dose long-term erythromycin therapy. Clin ORL 1992;85:1245-1252.
3. Haruna S, Oodori S, Tama I, et al. Eosinophilic paranasal sinusitis. ORL Tokyo 2001;44:195-201.
4. Chang YT, Fang SY. Tissue-specific immunoglobulin E in maxillary sinus mucosa of allergic fungal sinusitis. Rhinology 2008;46:226-230.
5. Gevaert P, Calus L, Van Zele T, et al. Omalizumab is effective in allergic patients with nasal polyps and asthma. J Allergy 2013;13:110-106.
6. Ota Y, Yamada C, Takazawa K, Rikitake A. Four cases of eosinophilic sinusitis that were administered omalizumab (Xolair®). Clin ORL 2012;105:1101-1106.
7. Tsurumaru H. Lymphoid follicle formation in sinus mucosa of chronic sinusitis. Jap ORL Soc 1996;99:1662-1675.
8. Sakuma Y, Ishitoya J, Komatsu M. New clinical diagnostic criteria for eosinophilic chronic rhinosinusitis. Auris Nasus Larynx 2011;38:583-588.
9. Matsuwaki W, Ookushi T, Asaka D. Chronic rhinosinusitis: risk factors for the reccurence of chronic rhinosimusitis based on 5-year follow-up after endoscopic sinus surgery. Int Arch Allergy Immunol 2008;146:7-81.
10. Jafec BW. Ultrastructure of human nasal mucosa. Laryngoscope 1983;93:1576-1599.
11. Balogh K and Pantanowitz L. Mouth, nose, and paranasal sonus. In: Mills SE (Ed.), Histology for Pathologists. pp. 403-432. Philadelphia, USA: Lippincott Williams and Wilkins 2007.
12. Djukanovic R, Wilson SJ, Kraft M, et al. Effects of treatment with anti-immunoglobulin E antibody omalizumab on airway inflammation in allergic asthma. Am J Respir Crit Care Med 2004;170:583-593.
13. Massanari M, Holgate ST, Busse WW, et al. Effect of omalizumab on peripheral blood eosinophilia in allergic asthma. Respir Med 2010;104:188-196.
14. Watanabe N, Owhashi M, Nawa Y. Clearance of passively transferred IgE antibody from peripheral blood of mast cell-deficient W/Wv mice. Int Arch Allergy Appl Immunol 1986;81:385-387.
15. Cotran RS. New roles for the endothelium in inflammation and immunity. Am J Pathol 1987;129:407-413.
16. Gevaert P, Holtappels G, Bachert C. Organization of secondary lymphoid tissue and local IgE formation to Staphylococcus aureus enterotoxins in nasal polyp tissue. Allergy 2005;60:71-79.
17. Bachert C, Zhang N. Chronic rhinosinusitis and asthma: novel understanding of the role of IgE 'above atopy'. J Intern Med 2012;272:133-143.

CHRONIC RHINOSINUSITIS ASSOCIATED WITH HYPER-IGE SYNDROME

T. Furukawa, Y. Takeda, H. Asao, N. Ohta, K. Futai, S. Kakehata

Department of Otorhinolaryngology and Head/Neck Surgery, Yamagata University School of Medicine, Japan

Abstract

The hyper-immunoglobulin E (hyper-IgE) syndrome is a primary immunodeficiency characterized by recurrent staphylococcal abscesses, recurrent cyst-forming pneumonia, and an elevated serum IgE level of > 2000 IU/ml. We present a – to our knowledge rare – case of an association between hyper-IgE syndrome and chronic rhinosinusitis in a 34-year-old woman. Endoscopic sinus surgery was performed on both sides to control the recurrent sinus infections. Ten months after surgery, no sinusitis flare-ups have been confirmed. Patients with hyper-IgE show abnormal STAT-3 activity. However, STAT-3 phosphorylation (STAT-3 activation) is not defective, and mutations that cause inhibition of STAT-3 nuclear import (DNA binding) have been observed. We examined her immunological background using her blood. Also, in our patient, it was considered unlikely that the level of STAT-3 phosphorylation clearly differs from that of a healthy individual under any stimulation conditions. On the other hand, the phagocytic ability of neutrophils was lower. These results suggested that patients with hyper-IgE exhibit an imbalance between humoral and cell-mediated immunity, in that immune response is predominantly humoral. Moreover, a decline in cell-mediated immune function may manifest as the decreased phagocytic activity of neutrophils.

Address for correspondence: Dr. Takatoshi Furukawa, Department of Otolaryngology, Head and Neck Surgery, Yamagata University Faculty of Medicine, 2-2-2 Iida-Nishi, Yamagata 990-9585, Japan. E-mail: t-furukawa@med.id.yamagata-u.ac.jp

Recent Advances in Rhinosinusitis and Nasal Polyposis, p. 165
Edited by Hideyuki Kawauchi, Desiderio Passali, Ranko Mladina, Andrey Lopatin and Dmytro Zabolotnyi
2015 © Kugler Publications, Amsterdam, The Netherlands

EFFICACY OF ENDOSCOPIC SINUS SURGERY-BASED ON MULTIDISCIPLINARY TREATMENT FOR CHRONIC RHINOSINUSITIS WITH BRONCHIAL ASTHMA

Nobuo Ohta, Yusuke Suzuki, Kazuya Kurakami, Takatoshi Furukawa, Toshinori Kubota, Yasuhiro Abe, Masaru Aoyagi, Seiji Kakehata

Department of Otolaryngology, Head and Neck Surgery, Yamagata University Faculty of Medicine, Yamagata, Japan

Conflicts of interests: none.
Funding: none.
Keywords: endoscopic sinus surgery, chronic rhinosinusitis, bronchial asthma

Abstract

Background: There is growing evidence that chronic rhinosinusitis (CRS) may be associated with bronchial asthma and recent reports suggest the effectiveness of endoscopic sinus surgery (ESS) in CRS patients with bronchial asthma. Whether ESS has a positive effect on the clinical course of asthma is still not clear. To clarify this point, the outcomes of ESS on asthma in patients with CRS were examined.
Subjects and methods: We performed a study to evaluate the effectiveness of ESS in twenty four CRS patients with bronchial asthma. The changes in symptoms, medication use and pulmonary functions in CRS patients with bronchial asthma before and after ESS were evaluated.
Results: There was an improvement in the asthma control score (wheeze, cough and shortness of breath), asthma medication use and pulmonary functions after ESS. **Conclusions:** This study provides corroborative subjective and objective evidence that ESS is feasible and effective in the management of CRS with bronchial asthma.

Address for correspondence: Dr. Nobuo Ohta, Department of Otolaryngology, Head and Neck Surgery, Yamagata University Faculty of Medicine, 2-2-2, Iida-nishi, Yamagata, 990-9585, Japan. E-mail: noohta@med.id.yamagata-u.ac.jp

Recent Advances in Rhinosinusitis and Nasal Polyposis, pp. 167-172
Edited by Hideyuki Kawauchi, Desiderio Passali, Ranko Mladina, Andrey Lopatin and Dmytro Zabolotnyi
2015 © Kugler Publications, Amsterdam, The Netherlands

Introduction

Chronic rhinosinusitis (CRS) is a common disease and a significant health problem. Although the medical and endoscopic sinus surgery (ESS) treatments for CRS have improved the symptoms of patients markedly, a subgroup of patients with CRS shows very poor response to all kinds of treatment modalities.[1] Bronchial asthma is a disease characterized by variable and reversible airway obstruction and considered to be one of the important factors for refractory CRS. The impact of ESS on bronchial asthma is still not controversial and bronchial asthma has been reported as improved, unchanged, and deteriorated after ESS in various studies.[1-4] To clarify this point, this prospective study was performed to evaluate the effect of ESS-based on multidisciplinary treatment for CRS with bronchial asthma.

Subjects and methods

Twenty-four CRS patients with bronchial asthma were enrolled in this study. Clinical characteristics of these patients were shown in Table 1. All CRS patients with bronchial asthma had nasal polyps and four patients had aspirin intolerance. All CRS patients with bronchial asthma underwent ESS under general anesthesia. The conditions of bronchial asthma in all the enrolled patients were evaluated before and after ESS. The study compares changes in symptom scores with objective measures of pulmonary functions in CRS patients with bronchial asthma before and after ESS. Inclusion criteria of the study were: 1) Age above 20 years; 2) Patients with medically refractory CRS at the time of ESS; 3) No underlying immunodeficiencies, cystic fibrosis or neoplasia. ENT surgeons evaluated patients every month before and after surgery for a period of 12 months for bronchial asthma. The physician's evaluation consisted of assessment of symptoms, physical examination, use of medication, and pulmonary function tests. Postoperatively, the ENT surgeons and physician routinely performed surveillance for recurrent disease, recurrent polyposis, CRS and asthma control. The subjective assessment was carried out by evaluating common symptoms of asthma (cough, shortness of breath and wheeze), medication use and QOL with asthma control test questionnaire. Bronchial asthma status was graded as well-controlled, partial controlled and lack of control, and the change in symptom score before and after ESS was analyzed. The CRS patients with bronchial asthma were on medical treatment for asthma with β2-agonist, theophyline derivatives, mast cell stabilizers and inhaled steroids. Objective lower airway evaluation was performed by pulmonary function tests which included forced expiratory volume in one second (FEV_1) and % predicted forced expiratory volume in one second (FEV_1 %), forced vital capacity (FVC), peak expiratory flow rate (PEF), V_{25} and V_{50}. Statistical analysis was performed using SPSS (Ver10). Paired t-test was performed to compare pre and post-ESS variables. A p value of < 0.05 was considered significant.

Table 1. Clinical characteristics.

Age, yr	41 (27-71)
Male/female	10/14
Course, yr	3.6 (0.5-6.5)
Polyps, no (%)	24 (100)
AR, no (%)	21 (90)
Aspirin intolerance, no (%)	4 (20)
Surgery history, no (%)	4 (20)

AR: allergic rhinitis

Results

Our study consisted of ten males and 14 females of the age group 27-71 years. The patients were diagnosed cases of asthma with medically resistant CRS on asthma medication of bronchodilators and steroids. We evaluated three basic symptoms of asthma; shortness of breath, wheeze and dry cough in these patients six months before and after ESS. On analysis of symptoms before ESS, three (12.5%) patients had well-controlled condition, 20 (83.3%) patients had partial control and one (74%) patient had uncontrolled situation. After ESS, there was a definite and statistically significant improvement in the number of symptomatic patients (Table 2). Objective assessment by pulmonary function test also demonstrated an improvement of scores after ESS. There was no significant difference in FEV_1, FEV_1 %, PEF, V_{25} and V_{50} values between before and after ESS. The FVC improved from an average of 3.54 preoperatively to 3.79 after ESS at the time of follow-up (Table 3).

Table 2. Asthma control grade.

	No	Well-controlled	Partial control	Lack of control
Preoperative	24	3 (12.5)	20 (83.3)	1 (4.2)
Postoperative	24	14 (58.4)	10 (41.6)	0

Data are presented as n (%). Likelihood $x^2 = 1.233$; p = 0.034

Table 3. Pulmonary functions.

	Preoperative	Postoperative
FEV_1	2.56 ± 0.46	2.63 ± 0.37
FEV_1 %	71.09 ± 4.05	69.68 ± 3.01
FVC	3.54 ± 0.46	3.79 ± 0.43*
PEF	6.96 ± 0.91	6.85 ± 0.9
V_{25}	0.73 ± 0.32	0.82 ± 0.19
V_{50}	2.47 ± 0.81	2.41 ± 0.65
V_{25}/V_{50}	4.45 ± 0.69	4.67 ± 0.42

FEV_1: forced expiratory volume in 1 second (FEV_1); FEV_1 %: % predicted forced expiratory volume in 1 second; FVC: forced vital capacity, PEF: peak expiratory flow rate. Paired t-test was performed to compare pre and post-ESS variables. p value of < 0.05 was considered significant.

Discussion

A spectrum of upper airway diseases, such as acute upper respiratory tract infection, nasal polyposis, allergic rhinitis and paranasal sinusitis can lead to or deteriorate chronic inflammation of the lower airways.[2,3] The rationale for treatment of the nose in asthmatic patients follows the concept of 'united airways', because nasal inflammation can influence the lower airways and intranasal corticosteroids can relieve symptoms of sinusitis and asthma.[4-6] ESS has been successfully used as a more feasible surgical approach to the treatment of medically refractory CRS.[5,6] Recent reports proposed the ideas explaining the underlying mechanism of 'united airway' as follows: 1) Sinonasal bronchial reflex, *i.e.*, a reflex bronchoconstriction by activation of a trigeminal afferent-vagal efferent neuralarc;[5] 2) Tissue eosinophils contribute to inflammation and injury of epithelium of the nose, sinuses and lungs;[6] 3) Silent dripping of infected material from the nose into the bronchial tree as a possible link between sinusitis and asthma; 4) Reduction in nitric oxide, which is a potent modulator of bronchial tone, a characteristic of CRS, may precipitate acute bronchial hyper-responsiveness.[5-7] As demonstrated in several studies in coexistent sinusitis and asthma, a proper treatment of involved paranasal sinuses can significantly improve asthma symptoms.[7-9] Dejima *et al.* and Loehrl *et al.* evaluated 88 and 85 CRS patients with bronchial asthma and reported an improvement in subjective and objective symptoms of asthma, decreased use of bronchodilators and improvement of pulmonary functions.[8-12] In our study the symptoms of asthma (cough, wheeze and shortness of breath) had a definite improvement after ESS, however, the effect was comparatively lower in the patients who had severe symptoms as compared to those with mild and moderate symptoms. Recent meta analysis clearly demonstrated that the medication use including steroid inhalers for asthma showed a significant reduction after ESS and the patients with severe symptoms had extensive nasal polyposis preoperatively and developed recurrence for which they underwent revision surgery.[13,14] In our patients, the use of theophylines, leukotriene inhibitors and inhaled glucocorticoids showed a significant reduction after ESS respectively. The visits to the emergency room/casualty are a common occurrence in patients of asthma during disease exacerbations. These patients require intensive care during these attacks and these episodes are a marker of poor asthma control. These meta analysis also have shown reduction of these episodes after ESS.[13,14] Pulmonary function tests were commonly performed for objective analysis. Mean of the various spirometric parameters were calculated as % predicted for that patient for the height, age, weight and sex before and after ESS. Recent meta analysis also indicated that an improvement was seen in the values of FVC, FEV, and PEF in the CRS patients with bronchial asthma after ESS.[13,14] This study demonstrated that ESS-based multimodality treatment improved both the subjective and objective outcome of CRS patients with asthma. These results may allow us to speculate that CRS patients with bronchial asthma showed improvement following ESS in terms of their asthma control levels including asthmatic symptoms as well as their pulmonary function. Further studies are warranted to improve the long-term effect of CRS with asthma.

Conclusion

The rationale for treating the nose in asthmatic patients follows the concept of 'united airways', because nasal inflammation can influence the lower airways. This study provides corroborative subjective and objective evidence that ESS-based multidisciplinary treatment is feasible and effective in the management of CRS with bronchial asthma.

Acknowledgements

This work was supported by the Ministry of Health, Labor, and Welfare of Japan. We express our sincere thanks to Mrs. Yuko Ohta, Uyo Gakuen college, for her editorial assistance.

References

1. Ishida A, Ohta N, Suzuki Y, et al. Expression of Pendrin and Periostin in Allergic rhinitis and Chronic Rhinosinusitis. Allergology Int 2012;61:589-595.
2. Ohta N, Ishida A, Kurakami K, et al. The Expressions and Roles of Periostin in Otolaryngological Diseases. Allergology Int 2014;63(2):171-180.
3. Van Zele T, Holtappels G, Gevaert P, Bachert C. Differences in initial immunoprofiles between recurrent and nonrecurrent chronic rhinosinusitis with nasal polyps. Am J Rhinol Allergy 2014;28:192-198.
4. Al Badaai Y, Valdés CJ, Samaha M. Outcomes and cost benefits of functional endoscopic sinus surgery in severely asthmatic patients with chronic rhinosinusitis. J Laryngol Otol;2014:128:512-517.
5. Benninger MS, Holy CE. The Impact of Endoscopic Sinus Surgery on Health Care Use in Patients with Respiratory Comorbidities. Otolaryngol Head Neck Surg 2014;151:508-515.
6. Grzegorzek T, Kolebacz B, Stryjewska-Makuch G, Kasperska-Zając A, Misiołek M. The influence of selected preoperative factors on the course of endoscopic surgery in patients with chronic rhinosinusitis. Adv Clin Exp Med 2014;23:69-78.
7. Bush CM, Jang DW, Champagne JP, Kountakis SE. Epidemiologic factors and surgical outcomes in patients with nasal polyposis and asthma. ORL J Otorhinolaryngol Relat Spec 2013;75:320-324.
8. Dejima K, Hama T, Miyazaki M, et al. A clinical study of endoscopic sinus surgery for sinusitis in patients with bronchial asthma. Int Arch Allergy Immunol 2005;138:97-104.
9. Loehrl TA, Ferre RM, Toohill RJ, Smith TL. Longterm asthma outcomes after endoscopic sinus surgery in aspirin triad patients. Am J Otolaryngol 2006;27:154-160.
10. Poetker DM, Mendolia-Loffredo S, Smith TL. Outcomes of endoscopic sinus surgery for chronic rhinosinusitis associated with sinonasal polyposis. Am J Rhinol 2007;21:84-88.
11. Kim SY, Park JH, Rhee CS, Chung JH, Kim JW. Does eosinophilic inflammation affect the outcome of endoscopic sinus surgery in chronic rhinosinusitis in Koreans? Am J Rhinol Allergy 2013;27:e166-169.

12. Batra PS, Tong L, Citardi MJ. Analysis of comorbidities and objective parameters in refractory chronic rhinosinusitis. Laryngoscope 2013;123 Suppl 7:S1-11.
13. Vashishta R, Soler ZM, Nguyen SA, Schlosser RJ. A systematic review and meta-analysis of asthma outcomes following endoscopic sinus surgery for chronic rhinosinusitis. Int Forum Allergy Rhinol 2013;3:788-794.
14. Georgalas C, Cornet M, Adriaensen G, et al. Evidence-based surgery for chronic rhinosinusitis with and without nasal polyps. Curr Allergy Asthma Rep 2014;14:427.

MAXILLARY SINUS DISEASE CAUSED BY DENTAL IMPLANTS – RADIOLOGICAL FINDINGS AND TREATMENTS

Nozomi Nomi, Satoru Kodama, Masashi Suzuki

Department of Otolaryngology, Oita University, Oita, Japan

Introduction

Odontogenic sinusitis is a well-recognized condition and accounts for approximately 10% of cases of maxillary sinusitis.[1] Sinusitis originating from an odontogenic source differs in its pathophysiology, microbiology, and management from sinusitis of other causes. Recently, many dentists perform dental implant surgery in dental hospitals. And consequently, the complications with dental implants have also increased. We report the radiological findings of odontogenic sinusitis caused by dental implants, which was successfully treated with endoscopic sinus surgery. A combination of a medical and surgical approach is generally required for the treatment of odontogenic sinusitis.

Case report

A 66-year-old man was referred to our department with a history of dental implant placement two years ago. His chief complaint was purulent rhinorrhea and nasal discharge due to opening from oral cavity to nasal cavity. Purulent rhinorrhea was shown in his right middle meatus and there was a fistula on maxillary alveolar process. Computed tomography (CT) of the paranasal sinus was performed, which revealed bone augmentation with implant insertion into the left maxillary sinus and soft tissue imaging with aberrant implant body and screws on the right maxillary sinus (Fig. 1).

Address for correspondence: Dr Nozomi Nomi, 1-1, Idaigaoka, Hasama-cho, Yufu-shi, Oita, 879-5593, Japan. E-mail: nnomi@oita-u.ac.jp.

Recent Advances in Rhinosinusitis and Nasal Polyposis, pp. 173-175
Edited by Hideyuki Kawauchi, Desiderio Passali, Ranko Mladina, Andrey Lopatin and Dmytro Zabolotnyi
2015 © Kugler Publications, Amsterdam, The Netherlands

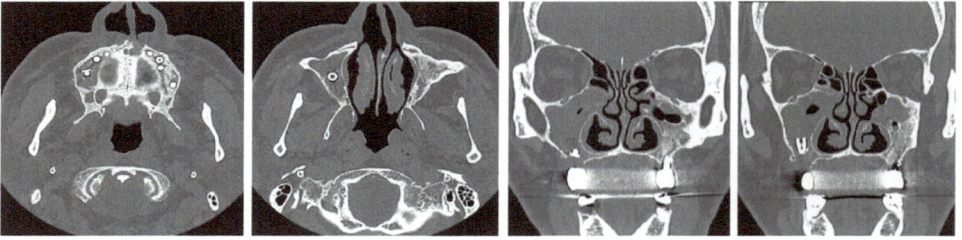

Fig. 1. Radiological exminations

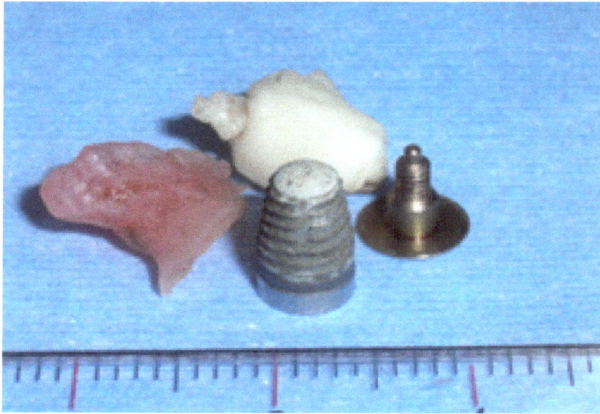

Fig. 2. Foreign bodies in the right maxillary sinus

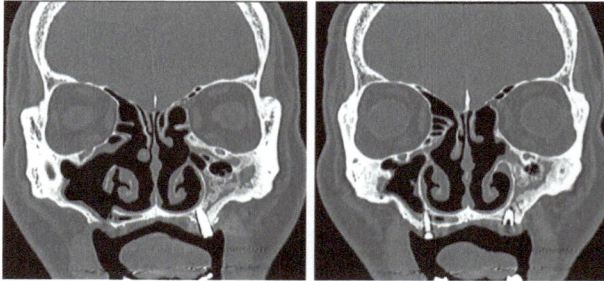

Fig. 3. Postoperative CT findings

Previously, he was treated with oral antibiotics for several months, however, his purulent rhinorrhea, nor his nasal discharge through oroantral fistula had improved. We thought that extraction of the foreign body and closing of the fistula were needed for improvement of the right maxillary sinusitis. We decided to perform endoscopic sinus surgery and removed aberrant implant bodies with an endoscopic procedure. We opened the bilateral maxillary and ethmoid sinuses. Intraoperative findings, mucoprulent discharge and polypoid mucosa were found in the right maxillary sinus and the left maxillary sinus was filled with granulation and bone augmentation. We removed foreign bodies (Fig. 2) and cleaned up the right maxillary sinus with saline. We also closed the oroantral fistula with a local mucosal flap. Pathological examination for the right maxillary mucosa revealed acute sinusitis. Bacterial examination of purulent nasal discharge on the right maxillary sinus revealed MRSA growth in the culture. Postoperatively, no oral antibiotics were needed except during the peri-operative period. One year after surgery, there is no recurrence of right maxillary sinusitis (Fig. 3).

Discussion

We report a case of odontogenic maxillary sinusitis caused by dental implantations. Odontogenic sinusitis usually occurs when the Schneidarian membrane is disrupted by conditions such as infections originating from the maxillary teeth, maxillary dental trauma, odontogenic pathology of the maxillary bone, or iatrogenic causes such as dental extractions, maxillary osteotomies in orthognathic surgery, and placement of dental implants.[1,2] Odontogenic sinusitis caused by dental implant placement shows a variety of symptoms and radiological findings. And the treatment of sinusitis of an odontogenic source often requires management of the sinus infection as well the odontogenic origin.

The association between an odontogenic condition and maxillary sinusitis requires a thorough dental examination of patients with sinusitis. Concomitant management of the dental origin and the associated sinusitis will ensure complete resolution of the infection and may prevent recurrences and complications. A combination of a medical and surgical approach is generally required for the treatment of odontogenic sinusitis. Recently, some otolaryngologists treated endoscopically,[1,3] however, it is still controversial whether implant removal is necessary or not for the treatment of odontogenic sinusitis caused by dental implant placement. In this case, we successfully treated odontogenic maxillary sinusitis with an endoscopic procedure without implant removal. Otolaryngologists and dentists should work together for diagnosis and treatment. Endoscopic sinus surgery might be indicated for intractable odontogenic sinusitis caused by dental implants.

References

1. Itzhak Brook. Sinusitis of odontogenic origin. Otolaryngol Head Neck Surg 2006;35:349-355.
2. Kretzschmar DP, Kretzschmar JL. Rhinosinusitis. Review from a dental perspective. Oral Surg Oral Med Oral Pathol Oral Radiol Endod 2003;96:128-135.
3. Lopatin A, Sysolyatin SP, Sysolyatin PG, et al. Chronic maxillary sinusitis of dental origin: is external surgical approach mandatory? Laryngoscope 2002;112:1056-1059.

PRESENCE OF HUMAN PAPILLOMAVIRUS AND IMMUNOHISTOCHEMICAL EXPRESSION OF CELL CYCLE PROTEINS P16^{INK4A}, PRB, AND P53 IN SINONASAL DISEASES

Zeyi Deng[1,2], Masahiro Hasegawa[1], and Mikio Suzuki[1]

[1]Department of Otorhinolaryngology, Head and Neck Surgery, Graduate School of Medicine, University of the Ryukyus, Okinawa, Japan; [2]Department of Otorhinolaryngology, Head and Neck Surgery, Zhujiang Hospital, Southern Medical University, Guangzhou, China

Objective

The aim of this study is to investigate the prevalence of human papillomavirus (HPV), and the relationship between HPV infection and expression of several cell cycle proteins, such as p16^{INK4a}, pRb, and p53, in sinonasal diseases.

Materials and methods

A total of 70 patients with sinonasal disease were taken into this study, including 32 cases with chronic rhinosinusitis (CRS), 17 with inverted papilloma (IP), five with IP associated with squamous cell carcinoma (IP-SCC), and 16 with primary sinonasal SCC. The presence of HPV DNA was detected by polymerase chain reaction (PCR) with two consensus primer sets, GP5+/GP6+ and MY11/MY09, and HPV subtypes were determined by direct sequencing. Expressions of p16^{INK4a}, pRb and p53 proteins were detected by immunohistochemistry (IHC). The IHC results were evaluated according to the extent of stained cells (p16^{INK4a} positive: more than 40% of stained cells; pRb or p53 positive: more than 25% of stained cells).

Address for correspondence: Prof. Dr. Mikio Suzuki, Professor and Head Department of Otorhinolaryngology, Head and Neck Surgery, University of the Ryukyus, 207 Uehara, Nishihara-cho, Okinawa, 903-0215, Japan. E-mail: suzuki@med.u-ryukyu.ac.jp

Recent Advances in Rhinosinusitis and Nasal Polyposis, pp. 177-178
Edited by Hideyuki Kawauchi, Desiderio Passali, Ranko Mladina, Andrey Lopatin and Dmytro Zabolotnyi
2015 © Kugler Publications, Amsterdam, The Netherlands

Results

The presence of HPV DNA was detected in two of 32 patients with CRS (6.3%), five of 17 patients with IP (29.4%), four of 16 patients with SCC (25.0%) and two of five patients with IP associated with SCC (40%), respectively. High-risk HPV-16 was the most frequently encountered subtype (10/13, 76.9%), followed by HPV-33 (two cases in IP) and HPV-18 (one case in SCC without IP). pRb positive was found in 78.1% (25/32) of CRS, 35.3% (6/17) of IP, and 68.8% (11/16) of SCC, respectively. While 62.5% (10/16) of SCC showed p53 positive, no CRS cases and only 5.9% (1/17) of IP exhibited p53 positive. In addition, p53 positive was observed in two of four SCC with HPV and eight of 12 SCC without HPV, respectively. Despite of HPV status, p16^{INK4a} positive was frequently detected in IP (82.4%, 14/17; four of five with HPV vs. ten of 12 without HPV), compared with only 12.5% (2/16) patients with SCC and none of CRS cases. Interestingly, when comparing the pRb staining with HPV status, SCC patients could be stratified as follows: HPV+/pRb+, one (6.3%); HPV+/pRb-, three (18.8%); HPV-/pRb+, ten (62.5%) and HPV-/pRb, two (12.5%). Statistical analysis revealed HPV DNA presence correlated with pRb negative ($P = 0.029$). A similar result was observed in IP samples. Thus, all five IP cases with HPV showed pRb negative, while six of 12 IP without HPV showed pRb positive ($P = 0.049$). In either IP cohort or SCC cohort, no correlations were found between HPV presence and p53 immunostaining, and between HPV presence and p16 expression.

Conclusions

Our findings indicate that sinonasal tumors, including benign IPs, IPs associated with SCC, and SCC, might be infected by HPV. An inverse correlation between HPV presence and positive pRb immunostaining was found in sinonasal IPs and SCCs. P16INK4a is not a reliable surrogate marker for HPV infection in sinonasal IPs.

SURGICAL MANAGEMENT OF INVERTED PAPILLOMA INVOLVING THE FRONTAL SINUS

Nobuo Ohta[1], Yusuke Suzuki[1], Kazuya Kurakami[1], Takatoshi Furukawa[1], Toshinori Kubota[1], Yasuyuki Hinohira[2], Yasuhiro Abe[1], Kazunori Futai[1], Masaru Aoyagi[1], Seiji Kakehata[1]

[1]Department of Otolaryngology, Head and Neck Surgery, Yamagata University Faculty of Medicine, Yamagata, Japan; [2]Department of Otorhinolaryngology, School of Medicine, Showa University Japan

Abstract

Inverted papilloma is a benign locally aggressive tumor in the nasal cavity and paranasal sinuses. Traditionally, inverted papilloma has been managed with external surgical approaches. However, advances in imaging guidance system, surgical instrumentation and intraoperative visualization have led to a gradual shift from external approaches to endonasal attachment-oriented surgery. We present seven cases of inverted papilloma involving frontal sinuses successfully removed by endoscopic median drainage (Draf III procedure) under endoscopic guidance without any additional external approach. The whole cavity of the frontal sinuses was easily inspected at the end of the procedure. No early or late complications were observed. No recurrence was identified after a follow-up period of an average of 39.5 months. Management of inverted papilloma extending to frontal sinus with the endoscopic median drainage approach is feasible and seems to be effective.

Introduction

Inverted papilloma is a common benign tumor of the nasal cavity and paranasal sinuses. The management of sinonasal inverted papilloma is often complicated

Address for correspondence: Dr. Nobuo Ohta, Department of Otolaryngology, Head and Neck Surgery, Yamagata University Faculty of Medicine, 2-2-2, Iida-nishi, Yamagata, 990-9585, Japan. E-mail: noohta@med.id.yamagata-u.ac.jp

Recent Advances in Rhinosinusitis and Nasal Polyposis, pp. 179-185
Edited by Hideyuki Kawauchi, Desiderio Passali, Ranko Mladina, Andrey Lopatin and Dmytro Zabolotnyi
2015 © Kugler Publications, Amsterdam, The Netherlands

due to its local aggressiveness, high recurrence rate, and malignant trasforma-
tion.[1] The incidence of its association with malignancy has been reported 1% to
5%.[2,3] The most common attachment site of the tumor origin is the lateral wall
of the nasal cavity.[1-3] The standard treatment strategy of inverted papilloma has
been complete wide local resection with external approach; however, incomplete removal of the attachment site is known to be the reason for recurrence
of the tumor.[3,4] The recurrence rate ranges between 0 and 60% depending on
the approach used.[2-4]

Several external surgical procedures, including Denker, medial maxillectomy,
lateral rhinotomy, osteoplastic flap procedure, and midfacial degloving approach
have been performed for advanced cases. Endoscopic removal of benign tumors
of paranasal sinuses has become more popular recently.[5-8] Advances in images,
surgical instrumentation, intraoperative navigation system, and angled visualization have led to a gradual shift from external approaches to endoscopic surgery.
However, endoscopic surgery of inverted papilloma extending to the frontal
sinus(es) is still challenging because of the narrow working space, angulated,
anatomically variable frontal recess and its proximity to the olfactory fossa
and anterior skull base. In the literature, there are limited reports presenting
series of patients with inverted papilloma extending to the frontal sinus treated
endoscopically.[1-6] We present seven patients with inverted papilloma involving
the frontal sinus successfully treated with the combination Draf III approach
(median drainage) and endoscopic medial maxillectomy. The aim of this study
is to present our experience in management of inverted papilloma extending to
the frontal sinus(es).

Subjects and methods

Patients

Seven consecutive patients with sinonasal inverted papilloma who attended
our department at Yamagata University Hospital, Yamagata, Japan, between
2008 and 2013 were enrolled in this study. The median age of these patients
was 58.4 years (range 38-79 years), with a median disease duration of 39.5
months (range, 19-54 months). Clinical features of the patients are shown in
Table 1. The diagnosis was made on the basis of clinical data, imaging, and
histopathologic findings.

Surgical methods

Two representative cases out of the seven we enrolled will be discussed here
more extensively and are shown in Figures 1 and 2. The first case (Case 1) is
a 44-year-old patient who presented with symptoms of chronic rhinosinusitis
without any history of previous sinus surgery. Rhinoscopy revealed a polypoid
grey mass in both nasal passages. Initial plain computed tomography (CT)

Table 1. Clinical characteristics.

Case	Age	Side	Symptoms	Attachment site(s)	Previous surgery	Stage	Outcomes
1	44 M	R	Obstruction	FR, ethmoid	0	T3b	recurrence (-)
2	67 M	R	Obstruction	FR, frontal	0	T3b	recurrence (-)
3	38 F	R	Obstruction	FR	2	T3b	recurrence (-)
4	54 F	L	Obstruction	FR, frontal	1	T3b	recurrence (-)
5	67 M	R	Obstruction	FR, ethmoid	1	T3b	recurrence (-)
6	79 F	R	Obstruction	ethmoid, frontal	0	T3b	recurrence (-)
7	60 M	R	Obstruction	ethmoid, frontal	1	T3b	recurrence (-)

M: male; F: female; R: right; L: left; FR: frontal recess; ethmoid: ethmoid sinus; frontal: frontal sinus; obstruction: nasal obstruction.

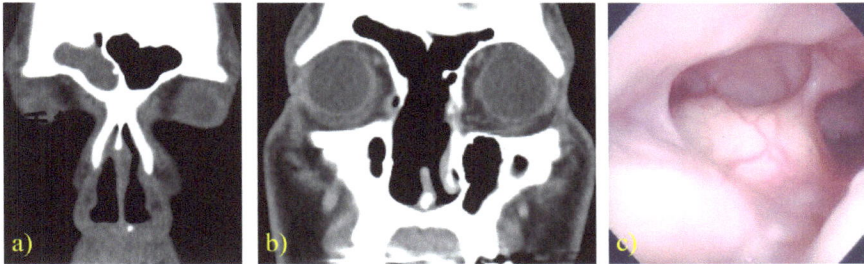

Fig. 1. a. Preoperative CT scan shows a soft tissue-density lesion in the right frontal sinus. b. One year postoperative, CT scan shows no soft tissue-density lesion in the right sinus. c. This endoscopic view shows the patient one year postoperatively with a nicely healed common opening into both frontal sinuses.

showed total opacification of the anterior and posterior ethmoids, frontal sinus and nasal cavity on the right side (Fig. 1 a). The tumor was removed under general anesthesia using a 0° and 70° scopes, shaver and curved diamond drill. After the lesion was debulked and removed from the nasal cavity and anterior ethmoids, bilateral full-house ethmoidectomy was performed. In the superior-anterior portion of the nasal septum the perforation filled with the mass of the tumor was visualized. No attachment to the edges of this perforation was seen. At this stage of the procedure it became clear that the site of origin of the lesion was located inside the right frontal sinus. The remaining part of the upper nasal septum was removed and the median drainage procedure was completed. The tumor origin was found on the lateral posterior wall of the sinus. The underlying bone was drilled down. The whole cavity of both frontal sinuses was easily inspected with the 0° and 70° scopes at the end of the procedure. Histopathology revealed inverted papilloma. One year postoperatively, endoscopic examination revealed thickening of the mucous membrane of the sinus with no signs of recurrence (Fig. 1 b and c).

The second representative case (Case 7) is a 60-year-old man with a history of recurrent inverted papilloma presented with signs of relapse of the tumor.

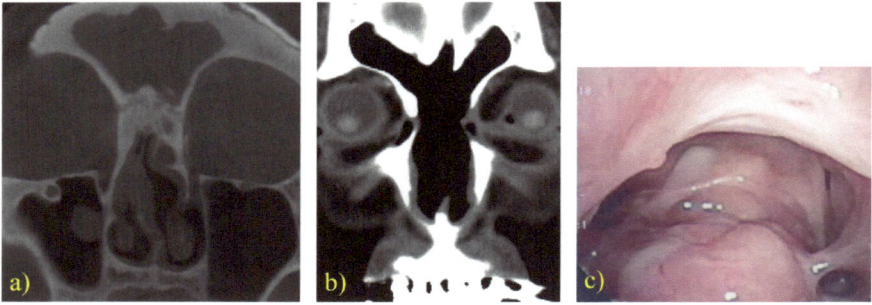

Fig. 2. a. Preoperative CT scan shows a soft tissue-density lesion in the right and left frontal sinuses. b. One year postoperative CT scan shows no soft tissue-density lesion in the right and left frontal sinus. c. This endoscopic view shows the patient one year postoperatively with a nicely healed common opening into both frontal sinuses.

He had previously undergone multiple polypectomies. After inverted papilloma was finally diagnosed, the right medial maxillectomy via the sublabial approach was performed. Four years after the last reoperation, endoscopy showed a whitish cauliflower-like mass bleeding on touch under the remnants of the bilateral middle turbinate. A biopsy was conducted and the recurrence of inverted papilloma was confirmed histopathologically. The CT showed total opacification of both frontal sinuses, lack of intersinus septum, presence of a low-density oval-shaped bony-like structure attached to the skull base at the level of the right anterior ethmoidal artery and marked thickening of the bone in the right olfactory groove with adjacent opacified ethmoid cell (Fig. 2 a). The median drainage (Draf III) procedure was performed under general anesthesia using 0° and 70° rigid scopes. After perforation of the upper part of the nasal septum the frontal sinus was entered in the midline and the bony bridges covering the right and left frontal recess were drilled down with a 0.5 mm diamond burr. The tumor was mobile, elastic, adherent to the mucosa of the upper part of the left frontal sinus mucosa. After exposure it was removed in two pieces. Postoperative endoscopic examination and CT performed one year after the procedure revealed no signs of relapse of the tumor (Fig. 2 b and c).

Discussion

Inverted papilloma involving the frontal sinus is rare and varies from 1.6% to 15% of cases of sinonasal inverted papilloma.[9-11] The importance of complete surgical resection is dictated by its locally aggressive nature, propensity for recurrence with incomplete resection, and potential to harbor malignancy. Due to the complex anatomy of the frontal sinus, high risk of complications and potential recurrence, a purely endoscopic approach has not been used routinely in cases of frontal sinus involvement. Traditionally, extended inverted papilloma involving the frontal sinus has been managed with Denker, medial maxillectomy, lateral rhinotomy, osteoplastic flap procedure, midfacial degloving approach, and a combination of open and endoscopic procedures. These methods, however, are associated with facial or gingival incision, external scar, loss of bony nasal or anterior maxillary support, infraorbital nerve paresthesia, postoperative facial swelling.

With the development of endoscopic surgical instrumentation it is possible to remove most sinonasal inverted papilloma with the attachment in the frontal recess, but rarely those originating from the sinus wall because of inadequate exposure.[11] The introduction of irrigated angulated burrs facilitated extended frontal sinus approaches such as Draf IIb and Draf III (median drainage). The Draf III procedure, also known as the modified endoscopic Lothrop procedure, enables visualization of the whole cavity of both frontal sinuses, which makes removal of the lesion originating from the frontal sinus feasible in most cases.[4,12] Efficacy of the endoscopic approach in inverted papilloma surgery was supported by a systemic review of the literature showing a low recurrence rate and low morbidity of this type of treatment.[8]

It is well recognized that most recurrences of sinonasal inverted papilloma result from incomplete removal of the attachment site, especially its bony component.[2] Radiological studies showed that in more than 90% of cases it is possible to identify the site of attachment of sinonasal inverted papilloma by the presence of focal bony thickening in high-resolution CT.[16] Magnetic resonance imaging (MRI) is useful to distinguish the border between mucus retention (hyperintense in T2 images) and the tumor. Preoperative planning based on high-resolution CT and MRI enables an endoscopic, tailored, attachment-oriented approach.[10] If the lesion is limited to the frontal recess and opacification of the frontal sinus is due to mucus retention, Draf IIa or IIb is the most convenient approach. However, if the origin of the tumor is located within the sinus or there is involvement of the contralateral side, probably the median drainage (Draf III) will be the most appropriate technique.

This procedure seems to be the most appropriate for endoscopic treatment of bilateral and/or multifocal frontal sinus lesions. Although intranasal surgery can be effective in most cases, some anatomical variants such as small antero-posterior dimension of the frontal recess can make it impossible.[17,18] Feasibility of intranasal radical removal of the inverted papilloma extending to frontal sinus can be adequately assessed preoperatively. In case of multifocal tumor or complications, the osteoplastic flap method may be needed. For this reason, all of the patients should be informed about the potential necessity of the osteoplastic flap method preoperatively.

In all cases of our study, while planning the procedure we expected multifocal involvement due to multiple previous procedures. Frontal recess is the most common attachment site of inverted papilloma extending to the frontal sinus. The advantages of the combination of median drainage and endoscopic medial maxillectomy are lack of external scarring, no infraorbital nerve paresthesia, shorter hospital stay, less postoperative pain, less postoperative facial swelling, less blood loss and low morbidity.

Conclusions

The results of present study that sinonasal inverted papilloma involving the frontal sinus can be effectively treated with the combination of median drainage procedure and endoscopic medial maxillectomy. The open approach is limited to cases with massive involvement of the frontal or supraorbital cell. The combination of median drainage and endoscopic medial maxillectomy avoids facial scar, and also provides better intraoperative visualization of the tumor's site of origin, and is associated with low surgical morbidity.

References

1. Kopelovich JC, Baker MS, Potash A. The Hybrid Lid Crease Approach to Address Lateral Frontal Sinus Disease With Orbital Extension. Ann Otol Rhinol Laryngol 2014; 123(12):826-830.
2. Krouse JH. Endoscopic treatment of inverted papilloma: safety and efficacy. Am J Otolaryngol 2001;22:87-99.
3. Pagella F, Pusateri A, Giourgos G, Tinelli C, Matti E. Evolution in the treatment of sinonasal inverted papilloma: pedicle-oriented endoscopic surgery. Am J Rhinol Allergy 2014;28(1):75-81.
4. Lund VJ, Stammberger H, Nicolai P, et al. European position paper on endoscopic management of tumors of the nose, paranasal sinuses and skull base. Rhinology Suppl 2010;22:1-143.
5. Gotlib T, Krzeski A, Held-Ziółkowska M, Niemczyk K. Endoscopic transnasal management of inverted papilloma involving frontal sinuses. Wideochir Inne Tech Malo Inwazyjne 2012;7(4):299-303.
6. Kamel RH, Abdel Fattah AF, Awad AG. Origin oriented management of inverted papilloma of the frontal sinus. Rhinology 2012;50(3):262-268.
7. Al-Qudah M, Graham SM. Modified osteoplastic flap approach for frontal sinus disease. Ann Otol Rhinol Laryngol 2012;121(3):192-196.
8. Busquets JM, Hwang PH. Endoscopic resection of sinonasal inverted papilloma: a meta-analysis. Otolaryngol Hesd Neck Surg 2006;134:476-482.
9. Walgama E, Ahn C, Batra PS. Surgical management of frontal sinus inverted papilloma: a systematic review. Laryngoscope 2012;122(6):1205-1209.
10. Zhang L, Han D, Wang C, et al. Endoscopic management of the inverted papilloma with the attachment to the frontal sinus drainage pathway. Acta Oto-Laryngol 2008;128:561-568.
11. Kim DY, Hong SL, Lee CH, et al. Inverted papilloma of the nasal cavity and paranasal sinuses: a Korean multicenter study. Laryngoscope 2012;122(3):487-494.
12. Wright EJ, Chernichenko N, Ocal E, et al. Benign inverted papilloma with intracranial extension: prognostic factors and outcomes. Skull Base Rep 2011;1(2):145-150.
13. Naidoo Y, Bassiouni A, Keen M, Wormald PJ. Long-term outcomes for the endoscopic modified Lothrop/Draf III procedure: a 10-year review. Laryngoscope 2014;24(1):43-49.
14. Carta F, Verillaud B, Herman P. Role of endoscopic approach in the management of inverted papilloma. Curr Opin Otolaryngol Head Neck Surg 2011;19(1):21-24.
15. Yoon B, Batra PS, Citardi MJ, Roh H. Frontal sinus inverted papilloma: surgical strategy based on the site of attachment. Am J Rhinol 2009;23:337-341.

16. Nakamaru Y, Fujima N, Takagi D, et al. Prediction of the Attachment Site of Sinonasal Inverted Papillomas by Preoperative Imaging. Ann Otol Rhinol Laryngol 2014;123(7):468-474.
17. Gotlib T, Niemczyk K, Balcerzak J, Krzeski A, Held-Ziółkowska M. Draf III procedures: the ENT Department, Medical University of Warsaw experience. Otolaryngol Pol 2010;64(7):40-43.
18. Farhat FT, Figueroa RE, Kountakis SE. Anatomic measurements for the endoscopic modified Lothrop procedure. Am J Rhino. 2005;19:293-296.

LONG-TERM MACROLIDE THERAPY FOR CHRONIC RHINOSINUSITIS: EVIDENCE OF EFFICACY?

Andrey Lopatin

Ear, Nose, and Throat (ENT) Clinic, Sechenov First Moscow State Medical University, Moscow, Russia

Chronic rhinosinusitis (CRS) is a complex condition that affects patient's quality of life and has profound effects on health care expenditure.[1,2] Management of this disease continues to challenge both patients and physicians. The aetiology and pathogenesis of CRS are still poorly understood. There is good evidence supporting the concept that inflammation, more than infection, is the dominant etiologic factor in CRS. Unlike acute rhinosinusitis, pathogenic microorganisms play a much smaller role in the pathogenesis of CRS.[3,4] Allergy seems to be a comorbid condition and not a primary factor in the development of CRS.[5]

At present, neither medical nor surgical treatment can ensure permanent control or enduring cure. As CRS is a chronic disease, concerns of medical treatment are related to the use of systemic agents over prolonged periods. Currently, the only proven treatment for control of CRS with polyps (CRSwNP) is topical nasal steroid sprays with or without systemic glucocorticosteroids (GCS). However, recurrent CRSwNP is not always prevented even with systemic GCS and the side effects can be serious, including cataracts and vertebral collapse.[6]

Oral antibiotics are the most common medication for CRS without polyps (CRSsNP)[7] and they are widely prescribed all over the world. Despite this, there is a surprising paucity of data regarding efficacy. Based on the available evidence, oral antibacterial antibiotics (only in case of acute exacerbation) and so-called 'long-term" courses of macrolide antibiotics are considered therapeutic options for CRSsNP.[8] The insufficient effectiveness of the standard courses of antibiotic therapy,[9] coupled with the doubtful benefit of GCS, especially

Address for correspondence: Andrey S. Lopatin, MD, Dr Med Sci., Partizanskayast. 33, bld 1, 55, 121351, Moscow, Russia.
E-mail: lopatin.andrey@inbox.ru

Recent Advances in Rhinosinusitis and Nasal Polyposis, pp. 187-192
Edited by Hideyuki Kawauchi, Desiderio Passali, Ranko Mladina, Andrey Lopatin
and Dmytro Zabolotnyi
2015 © Kugler Publications, Amsterdam, The Netherlands

in patients with CRSsNP without concomitant asthma and allergy,[10] and the inability to achieve 100% success with surgery[11] indicate the need to develop other treatment modalities.

Macrolide antibiotics have often been used in long-term therapy of CRS due to their anti-inflammatory effect similar to GCS. Knowledge of this dates back to a Japanese publication of long-term, low-dose macrolide treatment of diffuse panbronchiolitis, which also improved symptoms of concomitant CRS.[12,13] It seems that some non-antimicrobial properties of 14-membered (erythromycin, roxithromycin, clarithromycin) macrolides contribute to the success of therapy, namely their anti-inflammatory effect (inhibition of neutrophilic inflammation promoters such as interleukin-8), ability to modulate the immune response, to inhibit polyps' growth, to destroy biofilms, and to enhance protective properties of the respiratory tract mucosa.[14-17]

Several non-controlled and two placebo-controlled trials have studied the effect of long-term low-dose macrolide therapy on symptoms and quality of life in CRS patients. Results of the non-controlled investigations suggested good efficacy of this therapy in patients with recalcitrant CRS, particularly in cases where GCS and surgery failed to control the disease. However, results of the controlled studies were extremely controversial.

The first controlled study[18] assessed clinical efficacy of a 12-week course of roxithromycin (150 mg daily) in patients with CRSsNP. Statistically significant improvements in sino-nasal outcome test (SNOT-20) score, nasal endoscopy, saccharine transit time, and IL-8 levels in lavage fluid were identified in the macrolide group. Furthermore, the subgroup of nonatopic patients with IgE levels < 200 µg/L improved significantly more than patients with high IgE levels (> 200 µg/L). No improvement in any outcome was noted in the placebo-treated patients. However, statistically significant difference favoring the macrolide group at 12 weeks ($p < 0.01$) was only identified in terms of invalidated patients response scale. The authors did not report differences between study medication and placebo groups in SNOT-20 change scores and any objective measures. No improvements at all were not noted six weeks after cessation of a long-term course of roxithromycin treatment.

The second randomized controlled multicenter study[19] included patients both with and without nasal polyps unresponsive to medical and surgical treatment, half of them had asthma. Patients were treated with azithromycin (three days at 500 mg during the first week, followed by 500 mg per week for the next 11 weeks) or placebo. The study found no significant difference between azithromycin and placebo groups in the SNOT-22, patient response rating scale, VAS scores and SF-36, as well as nasal endoscopic scores, PNIF, and smell tests. However, patient response rating scale at the final endpoint three months after medication stop was significantly better in the azithromycin group. Interestingly, both controlled studies did not find an increase in macrolide resistant bacterial cultures from the middle meatus after a long-term low-dose course of macrolide therapy.

A meta-analysis performed later[20] summarized data of these two studies and compared SNOT scores at six, 12, and 24 weeks, calculating standardized mean differences. This analysis identified a statistically significant difference favoring macrolide therapy at 24 weeks (p = 0.03). However, with a standardized mean difference of -0.43 on the SNOT-20 (0-5 scale) equating to a 0.34 point decrease in SNOT score, this difference looks like clinically insignificant.

The discrepancy in these results may be explained by divergent CRS patterns, and macrolides have been found to be more effective in certain patients' populations. For instance, normal IgE levels are associated with a higher response rate to macrolide treatment versus elevated IgE levels.[18,21] In contrast, another prospective study demonstrated that an eight-week course of clarithromycin therapy was equally effective in both atopic and non-atopic patients with nasal polyposis.[22] Therefore, efficacy of long-term macrolides therapy looks evident in patients with CRSsNP, especially in those with low IgE levels, but the efficacy of macrolides in patients with CRSwNP has not been thoroughly studied yet.[5]

Our prospective randomized controlled study[23] was designed to evaluate the efficacy and safety of long-term courses (three and six months) of low-dose clarithromycin therapy in patients with CRSwNP after functional endoscopic sinus surgery (FESS). A total of 66 patients (36 men and 30 women) aged from 18 to 77 years with bilateral CRSwNP confirmed by endoscopy were recruited and randomly assigned to one of three study groups (22 patients per group) as follows: group 1 (clarithromycin 250 mg/day for 24 weeks); group 2 (clarithromycin 250 mg/day for 12 weeks); and group 3 (control, no antibiotic). All three groups received topical nasal steroid spray (mometasone furoate), 400 µg/day for 24 weeks after FESS. The majority of patients (79%) had at least one previous sinus surgery without long-term success (the mean number of surgeries was 3.2). After recruitment, all 66 patients underwent bilateral FESS performed by the same surgeon. Patients in group 1 and group 2 began long-term therapy with clarithromycin 250 mg/day on the first postoperative day and over 24 weeks (six months) or 12 weeks (three months), respectively.

Patients were carefully followed and seen at six weeks, 12 weeks, and 24 weeks after FESS. Results of treatment were based on evaluation of the following tests: 20-item SinoNasal Outcome Test (SNOT-20), 10-cm Visual Analogue Scale (VAS), olfactory 'Sniffin Sticks test', saccharin transit time test, endoscopic appearance score (EAS), active anterior rhinomanometry, acoustic rhinometry, and multislice computed tomography (CT). Additionally, eosinophil cationic protein (ECP) contents in the nasal discharge was measured and nasal swab for microbiological testing was collected from the middle nasal meatus prior to FESS at all postoperative visits. Skin prick tests for indoor and outdoor allergens were performed in all patients using standard methods. Final assessment of treatment results was carried out using the changes of EAS and Lund-Mackay CT scores at 24 weeks after FESS.

There were no significant differences between the three groups regarding age, sex, presence of atopy, severity of the disease, and number of previous

surgeries, as well as all the other initial parameters that we examined. Thirty-five patients had bronchial asthma, and 27 of these 35 patients presented with aspirin exacerbated respiratory disease. Atopy was confirmed by skin prick tests in 19 of the 66 initial patients

Treatment results were better for patients completing the course of long-term clarithromycin treatment in group 1 (antibiotic for 24 weeks) and group 2 (antibiotic for 12 weeks) compared to patients in group 3 (control no antibiotic). Statistically significant differences ($p < 0.05$) were obtained for all parameters (but not at every visit) between the study medication groups 1 and 2 and group 3 (control no antibiotics) with the only exception being for VAS and acoustic rhinometry where statistically significant evidence was not achieved.

The most remarkable results occurred in the evaluation of ECP concentration postoperatively. Before the surgery, median values of ECP concentrations in all three patients groups did not differ significantly, being 412.2 ± 123.1, 279.4 ± 85.9, and 330.8 ± 104.5, respectively. Six weeks after surgery, the ECP level in the nasal discharge increased in all study patients, being 553.2 ± 115.5, 604.0 ± 173.2, and 660.0 ± 171.6 ng/mL in groups 1, 2, and 3, respectively. Twelve weeks after FESS, a significant decrease of the ECP level in the nasal discharge was clearly observed in group 1 (antibiotic for 24 weeks): 153.6 ± 98.8 ng/mL ($p = 0.028$), and in group 2 (antibiotic for 12 weeks): 290.4 ± 77.2 ng/mL ($p = 0.036$). ECP level in the nasal discharge in group 3 (control no antibiotic) patients did not change significantly and was recorded as 654.0 ± 184.9 ng/mL ($p = 0.25$). Only in group 1 (antibiotic for 24 weeks) did the ECP concentration remain at the same low level (154.8 ± 89.8 ng/mL) at 24 weeks. In group 2 (antibiotic for 12 weeks) there was a slight increase of the ECP levels up to 338.1 ± 83.1 ng/mL when these patients were studied at 24 weeks (three months after stopping the antibiotics); however, with a p value of 0.084, the difference was not statistically significant. The mean ECP level in the nasal discharge in group 3 (control no antibiotics) rose significantly to 1000.0 ± 222.7 ng/mL ($p = 0.041$). It is important to note that the ECP level in patients treated with the macrolides over a full six months (group 1) was significantly lower than in those patients in group 2, who stopped the antibiotic therapy after three months of treatment.

Furthermore, the microbiological study of the swabs from the middle meatus revealed a wide spectrum of bacteria. In general, the number of clarithromycin-resistant strains (13%) remained constant throughout the course of clarithromycin treatment, agreeing with previous investigation that also failed to find resistant microorganisms after long-term treatment with low dose of a macrolide.[18,19,24]

The results of our study demonstrated the efficacy and relative safety of long-term low-dose macrolide (clarithromycin) therapy for preventing early recurrence of nasal polyps in patients with CRSwNP after FESS. Despite limited clinical data, our evidence suggests that patients with recurrent CRSwNP (surgical failures) deserve a trial of low-dose clarithromycin treatment (250 mg daily for three to six months), which may be initiated immediately after FESS along with maintenance therapy using topical nasal steroids.

References

1. Anand VK. Epidemiology and economic impact of rhinosinusitis. Ann Otol Rhinol Laryngol 2004;193:3-5.
2. Lund VJ. Impact of chronic rhinosinusitis on quality of life and health care expenditure. Clin Allergy Immunol 2007;20:15-24.
3. Brook I. The role of bacteria in chronic rhinosinusitis. Otolaryngol Clin North Am 2005;38:1171-1192.
4. Busaba NY, Siegel NS, Salman SD. Microbiology of chronic ethmoid sinusitis: Is this a bacterial illness? Am J Otolaryngol 2004;25:379-384.
5. Fokkens WJ, Lund VJ, Mullol J, et al. European Position Paper on Rhinosinusitis and Nasal Polyps 2012. Rhinology (Suppl) 2012;23:1-298.
6. Desrosiers MY, Kilty SJ. Treatment alternatives for chronic rhinosinusitis persisting after ESS: what to do when antibiotics, steroids and surgery fail. Rhinology 2008;46:3-14.
7. Fairbanks DN. Inflammatory diseases of the sinuses: bacteriology and antibiotics. Otolaryngol Clin North Am 1993;26(4):549-559.
8. Soler ZM, Oyer SL, Kern RC, et al. Antimicrobials and chronic rhinosinusitis with or without polyposis in adults: an evidenced-based review with recommendations. Int Forum Allergy Rhinol 2013;3:31-47.
9. Piromchai P, Thanaviratananich S, Laopaiboon M. Systemic antibiotics for chronic rhino-sinusitis without nasal polyps in adults. Cochrane Database Syst Rev 2011;(5):CD008233.
10. Parikh A, Scadding GK, Darby Y, Baker RC. Topical corticosteroids in chronic rhinosinusitis: a randomized, double-blind, placebo-controlled trial using fluticasone propionate aqueous nasal spray. Rhinology 2001;39:75-79.
11. Lund VJ. Evidence-based surgery in chronic rhinosinusitis. Acta Otolaryngol 2001;121:5-9.
12. Kudoh S, Uetake T, Hagiwara K, et al. Clinical effect of low-dose, long-term erythromycin chemotherapy on diffuse panbronchiolitis (English Abstract). Jpn J Thorac Dis 1984;25:632-642.
13. Nagai H, Shishido H, Yoneda R, et al. Long-term low-dose administration of erythromycin to patients with diffuse panbronchiolitis. Respiration 1991;58(3/4):145-149.
14. Hatipogulu U, Rubinstein I. Treatment of chronic rhinosinusitis with low-dose, long-term macrolide: an envolving paradigm. Curr Allergy Asthma Rep 2005;5:491-494.
15. Cervin A, Wallwork B. Macrolide therapy of chronic rhinosinusitis. Rhinology 2007;45:259-267.
16. Cervin A, Wallwork B, Mackay-Sim A, et al. Effects of long-term clarithromycin treatment on lavage-fluid markers of inflammation in chronic rhinosinusitis. Clin Physiol Funct Imaging. 2009;29:136-142.
17. Peric A, Vojvodic D, Matkovic-Jozin S. Effect of long-term, low-dose clarithromycin on T helper 2 cytokines, eosinophilic cationic protein and the 'regulated on activation, normal T cell expressed and secreted' chemokine in the nasal secretions of patients with nasal polyposis. J Laryngol Otol 2012;126:495-502.
18. Wallwork B, Coman W, Mackay-Sim A, et al. A double-blind, randomized, placebo-controlled trial of macrolide in the treatment of chronic rhinosinusitis. Laryngoscope 2006;116:189-193.
19. Videler WJ, Badia L, Harvey RJ, et al. Lack of efficacy of long-term, low-dose azithromycin in chronic rhinosinusitis: a randomized controlled trial. Allergy 2011;66:1457-1468.
20. Pynnonen MA, Venkatraman G, Davis G. Macrolide therapy for chronic rhinosinusitis: A meta-analysis. Otolaryngol Head Neck Surg 2013;148:366-373.
21. Haruna S, Shimada C, Ozawa M, et al. A study of poor responders for long-term, low-dose macrolide administration for chronic sinusitis. Rhinology 2009;47:66-71.
22. Peric A, Vojvodic D, Baletic N, et al. Influence of allergy on the immunomodulatory and clinical effects of long-term low-dose macrolide treatment of nasal polyposis. Biomed Pap Med Fac Univ Palacky Olomouc Czech Repub 2010;154:327-334.

23. Varvyanskaya A, Lopatin A. Efficacy of long-term low-dose macrolide therapy in preventing early recurrence of nasal polyps after endoscopic sinus surgery. Int Forum Allergy Rhinol 2014;4:533-541.
24. Cervin A, Kalm O, Sandkull P, Lindberg S. One-year low-dose erythromycin treatment of persistent chronic sinusitis after sinus surgery: clinical outcome and effects on mucociliary parameters and nasal nitric oxide. Otolaryngol Head Neck Surg 2002;126:481-489.

www.ingramcontent.com/pod-product-compliance
Lightning Source LLC
Chambersburg PA
CBHW040244230326
41458CB00104B/6475